ECG (

James H. O'Keefe, Jr., MD
Professor of Medicine, University of Missouri at Kansas City
Cardiologist, Mid-America Heart Institute
St. Lukes Hospital, Kansas City, Missouri

Stephen C. Hammill, MD
Professor of Medicine, Mayo Medical School
Director, Electrocardiography and Electrophysiology Laboratories
Mayo Clinic, Rochester, Minnesota

Mark S. Freed, MD
Cardiologist, President and Editor-in-Chief
Physicians' Press, Royal Oak, Michigan

Steven M. Pogwizd, MD
Associate Professor of Medicine
Attending Cardiologist, University of Illinois at Chicago
Chicago, Illinois

JONES AND BARTLETT PUBLISHERS
Sudbury, Massachusetts
BOSTON   TORONTO   LONDON   SINGAPORE

World Headquarters

Jones and Bartlett	Jones and Bartlett	Jones and Bartlett
Publishers	Publishers Canada	Publishers International
40 Tall Pine Drive	6339 Ormindale Way	Barb House, Barb Mews
Sudbury, MA 01776	Mississauga, Ontario	London W6 7PA
978-443-5000	L5V 1J2	United Kingdom
info@jbpub.com	Canada	
www.jbpub.com		

Jones and Bartlett's books and products are available through most bookstores and online booksellers. To contact Jones and Bartlett Publishers directly, call 800-832-0034, fax 978-443-8000, or visit our website www.jbpub.com.

Substantial discounts on bulk quantities of Jones and Bartlett's publications are available to corporations, professional associations, and other qualified organizations. For details and specific discount information, contact the special sales department at Jones and Bartlett via the above contact information or send an email to specialsales@jbpub.com.

The authors, editor, and publisher have made every effort to provide accurate information. However, they are not responsible for errors, omissions, or for any outcomes related to the use of the contents of this book and take no responsibility for the use of the products and procedures described. Treatments and side effects described in this book may not be applicable to all people; likewise, some people may require a dose or experience a side effect that is not described herein. Drugs and medical devices are discussed that may have limited availability controlled by the Food and Drug Administration (FDA) for use only in a research study or clinical trial. Research, clinical practice, and government regulations often change the accepted standard in this field. When consideration is being given for use of any drug in the clinical setting, the health care provider or reader is responsible for determining FDA status of the drug, reading the package insert, and reviewing prescribing information for the most up-to-date recommendations on dose, precautions, and contraindications, and determining the appropriate usage for the product. This is especially important in the case of drugs that are new or seldom used.

ISBN-13: 978-0-7637-8195-8

6048
Printed in the United States of America
12 11 10 09   10 9 8 7 6 5 4 3

Table of Contents

Abbreviations

APC	Atrial premature contraction	LBBB	Left bundle branch block
ASD	Atrial septal defect	LPFB	Left posterior fascicular block
AV	Atrioventricular		
AVNRT	AV nodal reentrant tachycardia	LVH	Left ventricular hypertrophy
		MI	Myocardial infarction
AVRT	AV reentrant tachycardia	MIN	Minute
BPM	Beats per minute	RBBB	Right bundle branch block
COPD	Chronic obstructive pulmonary disease	RVH	Right ventricular hypertrophy
ECG	Electrocardiogram	SA	Sinoatrial
HR	Heart rate	SEC	Second
HRS	Hours	SVT	Supraventricular tachycardia
IVCD	Intraventricular conduction disturbance	VA	Ventriculoatrial
		VF	Ventricular fibrillation
JPC	Junctional premature contraction	VPC	Ventricular premature contraction
LAFB	Left anterior fascicular block	VT	Ventricular tachycardia
		WPW	Wolff-Parkinson-White

Nomenclature

The relative amplitudes of the component waves of the QRS complex are described using small (lower case) and large (upper case) letters. For example: an "rS complex" describes a QRS with a small R wave and a large S wave; a "qRs complex" describes a QRS with a small Q wave, a large R wave, and a small S wave; and an "RSR' complex" describes a QRS with a large R wave, a large S wave, and a large secondary R wave (R'). When the QRS complex consists solely of a Q wave, a "QS" designation is used.

APPROACH TO
ECG INTERPRETATION

Each ECG should be read in a thorough and systematic fashion. It is important to be organized, compulsive, and strict in your application of the ECG criteria. Analyze the following 15 features on every ECG:

Once these features have been identified, ask the following questions:
1.   Is an arrhythmia or conduction disturbance present?
2.   Is chamber enlargement or hypertrophy present?
3.   Is ischemia, injury, or infarction present?
4.   Is a clinical disorder present (see item 14)?

Be sure to consider each ECG in the context of the clinical history. For example, diffuse ST segment elevation in a young asymptomatic patient without a previous cardiac history is likely to represent early repolarization abnormality, whereas the same finding in a patient with chest pain and a friction rub is likely to represent acute pericarditis.

1. Heart Rate

The following method can be used to determine heart rate. (Assumes a standard paper speed of 25 mm/sec)

Regular Rhythm

- Count the number of large boxes between P waves (atrial rate), R waves (ventricular rate), or pacer spikes (pacemaker rate)
- Beats per minute = 300 ÷ # large boxes

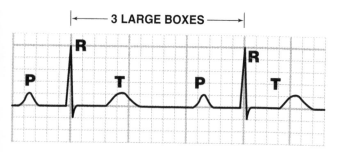

Heart Rate = 300 ÷ no. large boxes between "R" Waves = 300 ÷ 3 = 100 bpm

Note: It is easier to memorize the heart rates associated with each of the large boxes, rather than count the number of large boxes (1 ,2, 3, etc) and divide into 300:

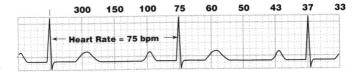

Note: If the number of large boxes is not a whole number, either estimate the rate (this is routine practice) or divide 1500 by the number of small boxes between P waves (atrial rate), R waves (ventricular rate), or pacer spikes (pacemaker rate):

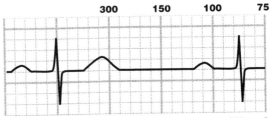

ESTIMATED Heart Rate = halfway between 100 and 75 = ~ 87 bpm (or 1500 ÷ 17.5 small boxes)

Note: For tachycardias, it is helpful to memorize the rates between 150 and 300 BPM:

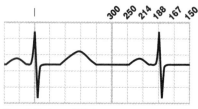

Heart Rate = 188 bpm

Slow or Irregular Rhythm

- Identify the 3-second markers at top or bottom of ECG tracing
- Count the number of QRS complexes (or P waves or pacer spikes) that appear in 6 seconds (i.e., two consecutive 3-second markers)
- Multiply by 10 to obtain rate in BPM

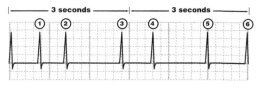

ESTIMATED Heart Rate = number of QRS complexes in 6 seconds x 10 = 6 x 10 = 60 bpm

2. P Wave

What It Represents: Electrical forces generated from atrial activation. The first and second halves of the P wave roughly correspond to right and left atrial activation, respectively.

What to Measure

- Duration (seconds): Measured from beginning to end of P wave.
- Amplitude (mm): Measured from baseline to top (or bottom) of P wave. Positive and negative deflections are determined separately. One small box = 1 mm on ECGs where 10 mm = 1 mV (standard)

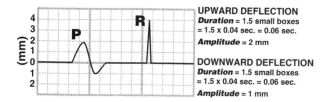

UPWARD DEFLECTION
Duration = 1.5 small boxes
= 1.5 x 0.04 sec. = 0.06 sec.
Amplitude = 2 mm

DOWNWARD DEFLECTION
Duration = 1.5 small boxes
= 1.5 x 0.04 sec. = 0.06 sec.
Amplitude = 1 mm

- Morphology:

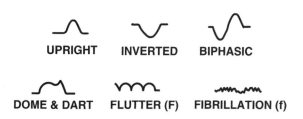

Normal P Wave Characteristics

Duration / Axis: 0.08 - 0.11 seconds / 0 - 75°

Morphology: Upright in I, II, aVF; upright or biphasic in III, aVL, V_1, V_2; small notching may be present

Amplitude: Limb leads: < 2.5 mm; V_1: positive deflection (< 1.5 mm and negative deflection < 1 mm

3. Origin of the Rhythm

Determining the origin of and identifying the rhythm is one of the most difficult and complex aspects of ECG interpretation (and one of the most common mistakes made by computer ECG interpretation programs). To determine the rhythm, several key features must be discerned and intergrated: heart rate, RR regularity, P wave morphology, PR interval, QRS width, and the P:QRS relationship. No single algorithm is able to simply describe all the various permutations; however the following rhythm-recognition tables, based initially on the P:QRS relationship and heart rate, provide a useful frame of reference:

P:QRS Relationships

P:QRS < 1: JPCs or VPCs; junctional or ventricular rhythms (escape, accelerated, tachycardia)

P:QRS = 1

- **P preceeds QRS**: Sinus rhythm; ectopic atrial rhythm; multifocal atrial tachycardia; wandering atrial pacemaker; SVT (sinus node reentry tachycardia, automatic atrial tachycardia); sinoatrial exit block, 2°; conducted APCs with any of the above

- **P follows QRS**; SVT (AV nodal reentry tachycardia, orthodromic SVT); junctional / ventricular rhythm with 1:1 retrograde atrial activation

No P Waves: Atrial fibrillation; atrial flutter; sinus arrest with junctional or ventricular escape rhythm; SVT (AV nodal reentry tachycardia, AV reentry tachycardia), junctional tachycardia or VT with P wave buried in QRS; VF

RATE < 100 BPM: Differential Diagnosis

Narrow QRS (< 0.12 sec) - Regular R-R
- **Sinus P‡; rate 60-100:** Sinus rhythm (item 2a)
- **Sinus P; rate < 60:** Sinus bradycardia (item 2c)
- **Nonsinus P; PR ≥ 0.12:** Ectopic atrial rhythm (item 2g)
- **Nonsinus P, PR < 0.12:** Junctional or low atrial rhythm (item 3d, 2g)
- **Sawtooth flutter waves:** Atrial flutter usually with 4:1 AV block (item 2x)
- **No P; rate < 60:** Junctional rhythm (item 3d)
- **No P; rate 60-100:** Accelerated junctional rhythm (item 3c)

Narrow QRS - Irregular R-R
- **Sinus P, P-P varying > 0.16 sec:** Sinus arrhythmia (item 2b)
- **Sinus and nonsinus P:** Wandering atrial pacemaker (item 2h)
- **Any regular rhythm** with 2°/ 3° AV block or premature beats
- **Fine or coarse baseline oscillations:** AFIB with slow ventricular response (item 2y)
- **Sawtooth flutter waves:** Atrial flutter usually with variable AV block (item 2x)
- **P:QRS ratio > 1:** 2° or 3° AV block or blocked APCs (items 6b-d, 2o)
- **P:QRS ratio < 1:** Junctional or ventricular premature beats or escape rhythm (items 3a, 3b, 4a, 4h)

Wide QRS (≥ 0.12 sec)
- **Sinus or nonsinus P:** Any supraventricular rhythm with a preexisting IVCD (e.g. bundle branch block) or aberrancy
- **No P†; rate < 60:** Idioventricular rhythm (item 4h)
- **No P†; rate 60-100:** Accelerated idioventricular rhythm (item 4g)

* Sinus P wave: Upright in I, II, aVF; inverted in AVR
† AV dissociation may be present

RATE > 100 BPM: Differential Diagnosis

Narrow QRS (< 0.12 sec) - Regular R-R

- **Sinus P*:** Sinus tachycardia (item 2d)
- **Flutter waves:** Atrial flutter (item 2x)
- **No P:** AV nodal reentrant tachycardia (AVNRT), junctional tachycardia
- **Short R-P (R-P < 50% of R-R interval):** AVNRT, orthodromic SVT (AVRT), atrial tachycardia with 1° AV block, junctional tachycardia with 1:1 retrograde atrial activation
- **Long R-P (R-P > 50% of R-R interval):** Atrial tachycardia, sinus node reentrant tachycardia, atypical AVNRT, orthodromic SVT with prolonged V-A conduction

Narrow QRS - Irregular R-R

- **Nonsinus P; > 3 morphologies:** Multifocal atrial tachycardia (item 2n)
- **Fine or coarse baseline oscillations:** Atrial fibrillation (item 2y)
- **Flutter waves:** Atrial flutter (item 2x)
- Any regular rhythm with 2°/3° AV block or premature beats

Wide QRS (≥ 0.12 sec)

- **Sinus or nonsinus P:** Any regular or irregular supraventricular rhythm with a preexisting IVCD or aberrancy
- **No P; rate 100-110:** Accelerated idioventricular rhythm (item 4g)
- **No P, rate 110-250:** VT (item 4f), SVT with aberrancy
- **Irregular, polymorphic, alternating polarity:** Torsade de Pointes (item 4j)
- **Chaotic irregular oscillations; no discrete QRS:** Ventricular fibrillation (item 4i)

* Sinus P wave: Upright in I, II, aVF; inverted in AVR

What it Represents

- PR interval: Conduction time from the onset of atrial depolarization to the onset of ventricular repolarization. It does not reflect conduction from the sinus node to the atrium.
- PR segment: Represents atrial repolarization.

How to Measure

- PR interval (seconds): From beginning of P wave to first deflection of QRS. Measure longest PR seen.

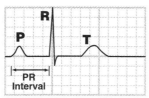

PR INTERVAL = 4 small boxes =
4 x 0.04 = 0.16 sec.

- PR segment (mm): Amount of elevation or depression compared to the TP segment (end of T wave to beginning of P wave).

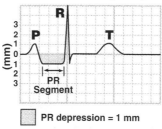

PR depression = 1 mm

Definitions

PR Interval

- Normal PR interval: 0.12 - 0.20 seconds
- Prolonged PR interval: > 0.20 seconds
- Short PR interval: < 0.12 seconds

PR Segment

- Normal PR segment: Usually isoelectric. May be displaced in a direction opposite to the P wave. Elevation usually < 0.5 mm; depression usually < 0.8 mm.
- PR segment elevation: Usually ≥ 0.5 mm
- PR segment depression: Usually ≥ 0.8 mm

5. QRS Duration

What it Represents

Duration of ventricular activation

How to Measure

In seconds, from the beginning to the end of the QRS (or QS) complex

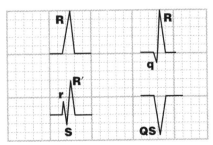

QRS duration = 1.5 small boxes = 0.06 sec.

Definitions

- Normal QRS duration: < 0.10 seconds
- Increased QRS duration: ≥ 0.10 seconds.

  <u>Note:</u> For the purposes of establishing a differential diagnosis, it is often useful to distinguish moderate prolongation of the QRS (0.10 to ≤ 0.12 seconds) from marked prolongation of the QRS (> 0.12 seconds)

6. QT Interval

What it Represents

Total duration of ventricular systole (depolarization [QRS] and repolarization [T wave])

How To Measure

- QT interval: In seconds, from the beginning of the QRS (or QS) complex to the end of the T wave. It is best use a lead with a large T wave and a distinct termination.

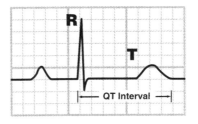

QT interval = 8 small boxes = 8 x 0.04 sec. = 0.32 sec.

- Corrected QT interval (QTc): Since the normal QT interval varies inversely with heart rate, the QTc, which corrects for heart rate, is usually determined

  ‣ QTc = QT interval divided by the square root of the preceding RR interval. **Example**: For heart rate of 50 bpm, RR interval = 1.2 seconds, and QTc = QT $\div \sqrt{1.2}$ = QT $\div$ 1.1

  ‣ Alternative method: Use 0.40 seconds as the normal QT interval for a heart rate of 70. For every 10 BPM change in heart rate above (or below) 70, subtract (or add) 0.02 seconds. The measured value should be within $\pm$ 0.035 seconds of the calculated normal. **Example**: For a HR of 100 BPM, the calculated "normal" QT interval = 0.40 seconds — (3 x 0.02 seconds) = 0.34 $\pm$ .035 seconds. For a HR of 50 BPM, the calculated "normal" QT interval = 0.40 seconds + (3 x 0.02 seconds) = 0.44 $\pm$ .035 seconds.

Definitions
- Normal QTc: 0.35 - 0.43 seconds for heart rates of 60-100 bpm. (The normal QT should be < 50% of the RR interval)
- Prolonged QTc: $\geq$ 0.44 seconds
- Short QTc: < 0.35 sec for heart rates of 60-100 bpm

7. QRS Axis

What It Represents
The major vector of ventricular activation

How to Determine
- Determine if "net QRS voltage" (upward minus downward QRS deflection) is positive (> 0) or negative (< 0) in leads I, II, aVF:

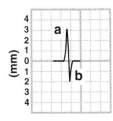

**NET QRS VOLTAGE =
upward – downward deflection (mm)
= a – b = 3 – 2 = 1 (positive)**

- Determine axis category according to the chart below:

Axis	Net QRS Voltage		
	Lead I	aVF	Lead II
Normal axis (0° to 90°)	+	+	
Normal variant (0° to -30°)	+	-	+
Left axis deviation (-30° to -90°)	+	-	-
Right axis deviation (> 90°)	-	+	
Right superior axis (-90° to +180°)	-	-	

+ = positive (> 0) net QRS voltage

- = negative (< 0) net QRS voltage

8. QRS Voltage

How to Measure

In millimeters, from baseline to peak of R wave (R wave voltage) or S wave (S wave voltage) (See QRS axis, previous page)

Definitions

- Normal voltage: Amplitude of the QRS has a wide range of normal limits, depending on the lead, age of the individual, and other factors
- Low voltage (from peak of R wave to peak of S wave): Limb leads: < 5 mm in all leads; precordial leads: < 10 mm in all leads
- Increased voltage: See LVH (item 10a), RVH (item 10c)

9. R Wave Progression

How to Identify

Determine the *precordial transition zone*, i.e., the lead with equal R and S wave voltage (R/S = 1)

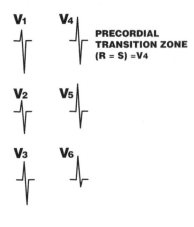

PRECORDIAL TRANSITION ZONE (R = S) =V4

Definitions

- Normal R wave progression: Transition zone = V_2-V_4; increasing R wave amplitude across the precordial leads (exception: R wave in V_5 often exceeds R wave in V_6)

- Poor R wave progression: Transition zone = V_5 or V_6

- Reverse R wave progression: Decreasing R wave amplitude across the precordial leads

10. Q Waves

How to Identify

A Q wave is present when the first deflection of the QRS is negative. If the QRS consists exclusively of a negative deflection, that defection is considered a Q wave, but the complex is referred to as a "QS" complex

What to Measure

Duration, in seconds, from beginning to end (i.e., when it returns to baseline) of Q wave. Note: When the QRS complex consists solely of a Q wave, a "QS" designation is used.

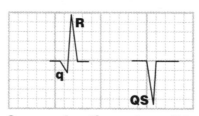

Q wave duration = 1 small box = 0.04 seconds

Definitions

- Normal Q waves: Small Q waves (duration < 0.03 seconds) are common in most leads except aVR, V_1 and V_2.
- Abnormal Q waves: Duration ≥ 0.04 seconds in leads III, aVL, aVF, and V_1; duration ≥ 0.03 seconds for all other leads

11. ST Segment

What it Represents

The ST segment represents the interval between the end of ventricular depolarization (QRS) and the beginning of repolarization (T wave). It is identified as the segment between the end of the QRS and the beginning of the T wave.

What to Identify

- Amount of elevation or depression, in millimeters, relative to the TP segment (end of T wave to beginning of P wave)

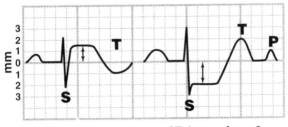

ST elevation = 1.5 mm   **ST depression = 2 mm**

- ST segment morphology

ST ELEVATION:

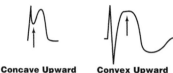

Concave Upward   **Convex Upward**

ST DEPRESSION:

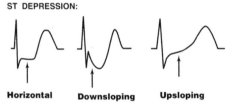

Horizontal   **Downsloping**   **Upsloping**

Definitions

- Normal ST segment: Usually isoelectric; may vary from 0.5 mm below to 1 mm above baseline in limb leads; in the precordial leads, up to 3 mm concave upward elevation may be seen (early repolarization, item 12a).

  Note: While some ST segment depression and elevation can be seen in normals, it may also indicate myocardial infarction, injury, or some other pathological process. It is especially important to consider the clinical presentation and compare to previous ECGs (if available) when ST segment depression or elevation is identified.

- Nonspecific ST segment: Slight (< 1 mm) ST segment depression or elevation.

12. T Wave

What it Represents

The electrical forces generated from ventricular repolarization

What to Identify

- Amplitude: In millimeters, from baseline to peak or valley of T wave:

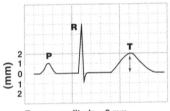

T wave amplitude = 2 mm

- Morphology:

UPRIGHT   PEAKED   INVERTED

NOTCHED   BIPHASIC

Definitions

- Normal T waves:

  Morphology: Upright in I, II, V_3-V_6; inverted in aVR, V_1; may be upright, flat or biphasic in III, aVL, aVF, V_1, V_2; T wave inversion may be present in V_1-V_3 in healthy young adults (juvenile T waves, item 12b)

  Amplitude: Usually < 6 mm in limb leads and ≤ 10 mm in precordial leads

- Tall T waves: Amplitude > 6 mm in limb leads or > 10 mm in precordial leads

- Nonspecific T waves: Flat or slightly inverted

13. U Wave

What it Represents

Controversial: Afterpotentials of ventricular muscle vs. repolarization of Pukinje fibers.

How to Identify

When present, the U wave manifests as a small (usually positive) deflection following the T wave. At faster heart rates, it may be superimposed on the preceeding T wave.

What to Determine

- Morphology: upright, inverted, or absent
- Height, in millimeters, from baseline to peak or valley

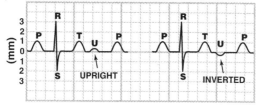

U wave amplitude = 0.3 mm

Definitions

- Normal U wave: Not always present; morphology: Upright in all leads except aVR; Amplitude: 5-25% the height of the T wave (usually < 1.5 mm); usually most prominent in V_2, V_3
- Prominent U wave: Amplitude > 1.5 mm

14. Pacemakers

Overview

Pacemakers are described by a 4 letter code:

▸ First letter: Refers to the chamber(s) <u>PACED</u> (**A**trial, **V**entricular, or **D**ual)

▸ Second letter: Refers to the chamber <u>SENSED</u> (**A, V** or **D**)

▸ Third letter: Refers to the pacemaker <u>MODE</u> (**I**nhibited, **T**riggered, **D**ual).

▸ Fourth letter: Refers to the presence (**R**) or absence (no letter) of <u>RATE RESPONSIVENESS</u>. Rate-responsive (or rate-adaptive) pacemakers can vary their rate in response to sensed motion or physiologic alterations (e.g., QT interval, temperature) produced by exercise by increasing their rate of pacing.

For example, a **VVIR** pacemaker PACES the Ventricle, SENSES the

Ventricle, ventricular pacing **INHIBITS** a sensed QRS complex, and is **R**ate responsive. A DDD pacemaker PACES and SENSES the atria and ventricle; the DUAL MODE indicates that sensed atrial activity will inhibit atrial output and trigger a ventricular output after a designated "AV interval," and that sensed ventricular activity will inhibit ventricular output and trigger atrial output.

▸ Typical single chamber pacemakers include VVI and AAI
▸ Typical dual chamber pacemakers include DVI and DDD

— Approach to Pacemaker Evaluation —

1. Assess underlying rhythm (100% paced vs. nonpaced intrinsic rhythm with pacemaker in demand mode)

- 100% ventricular paced

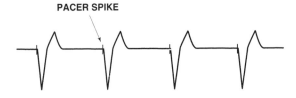

PACER SPIKE

- Ventricular pacing in <u>demand mode</u> (inconstant ventricular pacing from output inhibition by intrinsic sinus rhythm)

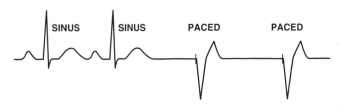

SINUS   SINUS   PACED   PACED

2. Determine the chamber(s) **PACED**

Determine relationship of pacing spike to P wave and QRS complex: A spike preceding the P wave typically represents atrial pacing; a spike preceding the QRS complex typically represents ventricular pacing.

- Atrial (A) paced beat

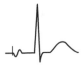

- Ventricular (V) paced beat

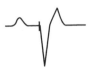

- Atrial (A) and ventricular (V) paced beat

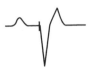

3. Determine timing intervals from 2 consecutively paced beats:

- For atrial pacing, determine the A-A interval

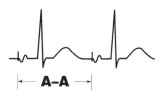

- For ventricular pacing, determine the V-V interval

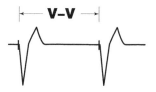

- For dual chamber pacing, determine the A-V and V-A intervals

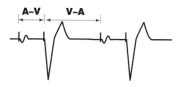

4. Determine the chamber(s) **SENSED**

- **Atrial pacemaker:** Proper atrial sensing is present when intrinsic atrial activation (native P wave) is always followed by 1) a native P wave that occurs at an interval less than the A-A interval; *or* 2) an atrial-paced beat that occurs after an interval equal to the A-A interval

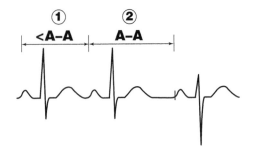

- **Ventricular pacemaker:** Proper ventricular sensing is present when intrinsic ventricular activation (native QRS complex) is always followed by: 1) a native QRS complex that occurs at an interval less than the V-V interval; *or* 2) a ventricular-paced beat that occurs after an interval equal to the V-V interval

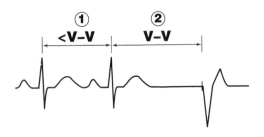

- **Dual chamber pacemaker:**
  - Atrial sensing is evident when intrinsic atrial activation (native P wave) is always followed by: 1) a native QRS complex that occurs at an interval less than the A-V interval; *or* 2) a ventricular-paced beat that occurs at an interval equal to the A-V interval

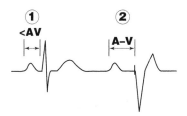

  - Ventricular sensing is evident when intrinsic ventricular activation (native QRS complex) is always followed by: 1) a native P wave that occurs at an interval less than the V-A interval; *or* 2) an atrial-paced beat that occurs at an interval equal to the V-A interval

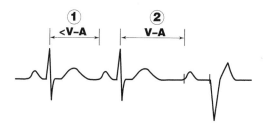

5. Determine the sequence of complexes representing normal pacing function. (Keep in mind that single chamber pacing on the surface ECG does not exclude the possibility that a dual chamber pacemaker is present — ventricular-paced beats may be due to a single chamber ventricular pacemaker or a dual chamber pacemaker in which ventricular spikes are timed to follow P waves [DDD pacemaker])

Pacing mode	Atrial pacing spike	Ventricular pacing spike
Atrial pacing	+	—
Ventricular pacing	—	+
Dual-chamber (DDD) pacing	+	+
	+	—
	—	+
	—	—

+   Pacing spike present on surface ECG
—   Pacing spike absent on surface ECG

6. Look for pacemaker malfunction

A. Failure to Capture (item 13f): Are any pacing spikes not followed by a depolarization?

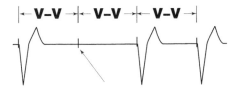

B. Sensing Abnormalities

- **Undersensing**: Based on timing intervals, are there pacing spikes that should have been inhibited by a native P wave or QRS complex but were not? This results in a paced beat that appears *EARLIER* than expected.

  ▸ Example: For ventricular pacing, undersensing is evident when a native QRS complex is followed by a ventricular-paced beat at an interval < V-V interval.

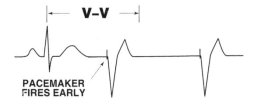

- **Oversensing**: Based on timing intervals, are there pacing spikes that should have been initiated after a native P wave or QRS complex but were not? This results in a paced beat that appears *LATER* than expected.

Examples:

▸ For ventricular pacing, oversensing occurs when a native QRS is followed by a ventricular-paced beat at an interval much greater than the V-V interval. Causes include:

- Oversensing of the T wave (item 13j), in which the T wave is sensed as (mistaken for) a QRS complex:

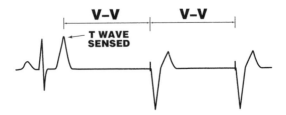

- Or muscle contractions (myopotential inhibition; item 13k), in which a myopotential is sensed as (mistaken for) a QRS complex:

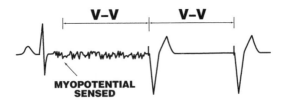

C. Others: Less common types of pacemaker malfunction include pacemaker not firing (item 13h), pacemaker slowing (item 13i), and pacemaker-mediated tachycardia (item 13m).

DIFFERENTIAL DIAGNOSIS

DIFFERENTIAL DIAGNOSIS

P Wave

— LEAD I —

Inverted P Wave

- Ectopic atrial beat (item 2i) or rhythm (item 2g)
- Junctional or ventricular rhythm with retrograde atrial activation (item 2t)
- Dextrocardia (item 14k): inverted P-QRS-T in leads I and aVL with *reverse* R wave progression in the precordial leads
- Reversal of right and left arm leads (item 1c): inverted P-QRS-T in leads I and aVL with *normal* R wave progression in the precordial leads

— LEAD II —

Tall Peaked P Wave

- Right atrial abnormality (item 8a)
- Biatrial abnormality (item 8d)

Bifid P Wave with Peak-to-Peak Interval < 0.03 Seconds

- Normal

Bifid P Wave with Peak-to-Peak Interval > 0.03 Seconds and P Wave Duration > 0.12 Seconds

- Left atrial abnormality (item 8b)

Inverted P Wave

- Ectopic atrial beat (item 2i) or rhythm (item 2g)
- Junctional or ventricular beats or rhythm with retrograde atrial activation (item 2t)

Sawtooth Regular P Waves

- Atrial flutter (item 2r)
- Tremor (e.g., Parkinson's disease) (item 1d)

Irregularly Irregular Baseline

- Atrial fibrillation (item 2s)
- Artifact due to tremor (item 1d)
- Multifocal atrial tachycardia (item 2n)

Multiple P Wave Morphologies

- Wandering atrial pacemaker (rate ≤ 100 bpm) (item 2h)
- Multifocal atrial tachycardia (rate > 100 bpm) (item 2n)
- Sinus or atrial rhythm with multiple APCs

— LEAD V$_1$ —

Tall Upright P Wave

- Right atrial abnormality (item 8a)

Deep Inverted P Waves

- Left atrial abnormality (item 8b)

Dome and Dart (p. 5)

- Ectopic atrial rhythm (item 2g)

— NO P WAVES —

P Waves Present but Hidden

- Ectopic atrial rhythm or APCs (P waves hidden in preceding T wave)
- Junctional rhythm or SVT (P wave buried in QRS)
- Supraventricular rhythm with marked first-degree AV block (P wave hidden in preceding T wave)

P Waves Not Present

- Sinoventricular conduction (hyperkalemia; item 14e)
- Marked sinoatrial exit block or sinus bradycardia with junctional or ventricular rhythm (escape or accelerated)
- Sinus arrest (item 2e)

PR Interval

Prolonged (> 0.20 seconds) PR Interval

- First-degree AV block (item 6a)
- Complete heart block (item 6e): PR interval varies and may intermittently exceed 0.20 seconds

- Supraventricular or junctional rhythm with retrograde atrial activation (item 2t): P wave inverted in lead II
- Atrial premature contraction (item 2i)

Short (< 0.12 seconds) PR Interval

- Short PR with sinus rhythm and normal QRS (item 6g)
- Wolff-Parkinson-White pattern (item 6h): delta wave, wide QRS, ST-T changes in a direction opposite to main deflection of QRS
- Low ectopic atrial rhythm (item 2g): usually > 0.11 seconds; P wave inverted in lead II
- Ectopic junctional beat or rhythm with retrograde atrial activation (item 2t): usually < 0.11 seconds; P wave inverted in lead II

PR Segment

PR Depression

- Normals: < 0.8 mm
- Pericarditis (item 14p)
- Pseudodepression due to atrial flutter (item 2r) or Parkinson's tremor (item 1d)
- Atrial infarction: reciprocal elevation in opposite leads; inferior MI usually evident

PR Elevation

- Normals: < 0.5 mm
- Pericarditis (item 14p): lead aVR only
- Atrial infarction: reciprocal depression in opposite leads

Increased (0.10 to < 0.12 seconds)

- Left anterior fascicular block (item 7c)
- Left posterior fascicular block (item 7d)
- Incomplete LBBB
- Incomplete RBBB (item 7a)
- Nonspecific IVCD (item 12c)
- LVH (item 10b)
- RVH (item 10c)
- Supraventricular beat or rhythm with aberrant intraventricular conduction (item 7i)
- Fusion beats (item 5a)
- WPW pattern (item 6h)
- VPCs originating near the bundle of His (i.e., high in the interventricular septum)

Increased (> 0.12 seconds)

- RBBB (item 7b)
- LBBB (item 7f)
- Supraventricular beat or rhythm with aberrant intraventricular conduction (item 7i)
- Fusion beats (item 5a)
- WPW pattern (item 6h)
- VPCs (item 4a)
- Ventricular rhythm
- Nonspecific IVCD (item 12c)
- Paced beat

QRS Amplitude

Low Voltage QRS

- Chronic lung disease (item 14m)
- Pericardial effusion (item 14o)
- Myxedema (item 14t)
- Obesity
- Pleural effusion
- Restrictive or Infiltrative cardiomyopathies
- Diffuse coronary disease

Tall QRS

- LVH (item 10a)
- LBBB (item 7f)
- WPW (item 6h)
- Normals with thin body habitus

Prominent R Wave in Lead V_1

- RVH (item 10c)
- Posterior wall MI (item 11l)
- Incorrect lead placement: electrode for lead V_1 placed in 3rd instead of 4th intercostal space
- Skeletal deformities (e.g., pectus excavatum)
- RBBB (item 7b)
- WPW (item 6h)
- Duchenne's muscular dystrophy

Alternation in Amplitude

- Electrical alternans (item 9e)

QRS Axis

Left Axis Deviation

- Left anterior fascicular block (if axis > -45°, item 7c)
- Inferior wall MI (item 11e, k)
- LBBB (item 7f)
- LVH (items 10 a, b)
- Ostium primum ASD (item 14j)
- COPD (item 14m)
- Hyperkalemia (item 14e)

Right Axis Deviation

- RVH (item 10c)
- Vertical heart
- COPD (item 14m)
- Pulmonary embolus (item 14n)
- Left posterior fascicular block (item 7d)
- Lateral wall MI (items 11d, j)
- Dextrocardia (item 14k)
- Lead reversal (item 1c)
- Ostium secundum ASD (item 14i)

Q Wave Myocardial Infarction (Item 11)

- Anterolateral MI: Q waves $\geq$ 0.03 seconds in V_4-V_6
- Anterior MI· Q waves $\geq$ 0.03 seconds in two of leads V_2-V_4 (or decreasing R wave amplitude in V_2-V_5)
- Anteroseptal MI: Q waves $\geq$ 0.04 seconds in V_1 and Q waves $\geq$ 0.03 seconds in V_2-V_3 (and sometimes V_4)
- Lateral/high lateral MI: Q wave $\geq$ 0.03 seconds in lead I and $\geq$ 0.04 in lead aVL
- Inferior MI: Q waves in at least two of leads II, III, and aVF (Q waves $\geq$ 0.03 seconds in II and $\geq$ 0.04 seconds in III and aVF)

Pseudoinfarcts (Q waves in absence of myocardial infarction)

- Wolff-Parkinson-White (item 6h)
- Hypertrophic cardiomyopathy (item 14q)
- LVH (items 10a, b)
- RVH (item 10c)
- Left anterior fascicular block (item 7c)
- COPD (item 14m)
- Amyloid heart (or other infiltrative diseases)
- Cardiomyopathy
- Chest deformity (e.g., pectus excavatum)
- Pulmonary embolism (item 14n)
- Myocarditis
- Hyperkalemia (14g)
- Lead reversal (item 1c)
- Corrected transposition

- Dextrocardia (item 14k)
- LBBB
- Pancreatitis
- Muscular dystrophy
- Mitral valve prolapse
- Myocardial contusion
- Left/right atrial enlargement: Prominent atrial repolarization wave (Ta) can depress the PR segment to mimic a Q wave
- Pneumothorax

R Wave Progression (Precordial Leads)

Early R Wave Progression (tall R wave in V_1, V_2; R/S > 1)

- RVH (item 10c)
- Posterior MI (item 11f)
- RBBB (item 7b)
- WPW (item 7h)
- Normals
- Duchenne's muscular dystrophy

Poor R Wave Progression (the first precordial lead where R wave amplitude $\geq$ S wave amplitude = V_5 or V_6)

- Normals (abnormal lead placement)
- Anteroseptal or anterior MI (items 11c, b)
- Dilated or hypertrophic cardiomyopathy
- LVH (item 10b)
- COPD (item 14m)
- Cor pulmonale (item 14n)

- RVH (item 10c)
- Left anterior fascicular block (item 7c)

Reverse R Wave Progression (decreasing R wave amplitude across precordial leads)
- Anterior MI (item 11b)
- Dextrocardia (item 14k)

QRS Morphology

Initial Slurring of R Wave (delta wave)
- WPW pattern (item 6h)

Terminal Notching (of R or S wave)
- Hypothermia (Osborne wave; item 14u)
- Early repolarization
- Pacemaker spike (failure to sense; item 13g)
- Atrial flutter (item 2r): Flutter waves may be superimposed on QRS

ST Segment

ST Elevation
- Myocardial injury (item 12e): Convex upward ST elevation localized to a *few* leads and ends with an inverted T (unless hyperacute); reciprocal ST depression evident in other leads; Q waves frequently present; ST & T wave changes *evolve*; T wave becomes inverted *before* ST segment back to baseline
- Acute pericarditis (item 14p): Widespread ST elevation (I-III, aVF,

V_3-V_6); *no reciprocal* ST depression in other leads except aVR; *no Q wave*; PR segment depression; ST & T wave changes evolve; T wave becomes inverted *after* ST segment back to baseline

- Ventricular aneurysm (item 11m): ST elevation usually with deep Q wave or QS in same leads; ST & T wave changes persist and are *stable* over a long period of time
- Early repolarization (item 12a): Concave upward ST elevation that ends with an upward T wave; notching on the downstroke of the R wave; large symmetric T waves; ST and T wave changes are *stable* over a long time period
- LVH (item 10b)
- Bundle branch block (items 7b, 7f)
- Central nervous system disease (item 14s)
- Apical hypertrophic cardiomyopathy (item 14q)
- Hyperkalemia (item 14e)
- Acute cor pulmonale (item 14n)
- Myocarditis
- Myocardial tumor

ST Depression

- Myocardial ischemia (item 12d): horizontal or downsloping
- Repolarization changes secondary to ventricular hypertrophy or IVCD (item 12g)
- Digitalis effect (item 14a)
- "Pseudodepression" due to superimposition of atrial flutter waves or prominent atrial repolarization wave (atrial enlargement, pericarditis, atrial infarction) on the ST segment
- Central nervous system disorder (item 14s)
- Hypokalemia (item 14f)
- Quinidine effect
- Mitral valve prolapse

Nonspecific ST Changes

- Organic heart disease
- Drugs (e.g., quinidine)
- Electrolyte disorders (e.g., hypokalemia, item 14f)
- Hyperventilation
- Hypothyroidism (item 14t)
- Stress
- Pancreatitis
- Pericarditis (item 14p)
- CNS disorders (item 14s)
- LVH (item 10b)
- RVH (item 10c)
- Bundle branch block (items 7a, f)
- Healthy adults (normal variant) (item 1b)

T Wave

Tall Peaked T Waves

- Acute MI (item 12e)
- Angina pectoris
- Normal variant (item 1b): usually effects mid-precordial leads
- Hyperkalemia (item 14e): more common when the rise in serum potassium is acute
- Intracranial bleeding (item 14s)
- LVH (item 10b)
- RVH (item 10c)

- LBBB (item 7f)
- Superimposed P wave: from APC, sinus rhythm with marked first-degree AV block, complete heart block, etc.
- Anemia

Deeply Inverted T Waves

- Myocardial ischemia (item 12d)
- LVH (items 10b and 12g)
- RVH (items 10c and 12g)
- Central nervous system disorder (item 14s)
- WPW (items 6h and 12g)

Nonspecific T Waves

- Persistent juvenile pattern: T wave inversion in V_1-V_3 in young adults
- Organic heart disease
- Drugs (e.g., quinidine)
- Electrolyte disorders (e.g., hypokalemia, item 14f)
- Hyperventilation
- Hypothyroidism (item 14t)
- Stress
- Pancreatitis
- Pericarditis (item 14p)
- CNS disorders (item 14s)
- LVH (item 10b)
- RVH (item 10c)
- Bundle branch block (items 7a, f)
- Healthy adults (normal variant) (item 1b)

Long QT Interval

- *Acquired conditions*
  - Drugs (quinidine, procainamide, disopyramide, amiodarone, sotalol, phenothiazine, tricyclics, lithium) (item 14c, d)
  - Hypomagnesemia
  - Hypocalcemia (item 14h)
  - Marked bradyarrhythmias
  - Intracranial hemorrhage (item 14s)
  - Myocarditis
  - Mitral valve prolapse
  - Hypothyroidism (item 14t)
  - Hypothermia (item 14u)
  - Liquid protein diets
- *Congenital disorders*
  - Romano-Ward syndrome (normal hearing)
  - Jervell and Lange-Nielson syndrome (deafness)

Short QT Interval

- Hypercalcemia (item 14g)
- Hyperkalemia (item 14e)
- Digitalis effect (item 14a)
- Acidosis
- Vagal stimulation
- Hyperthyroidism
- Hyperthermia

U Wave

Prominent U Wave

- Hypokalemia (item 14f)
- Bradyarrhythmias
- Hypothermia (item 14u)
- LVH (item 10b)
- Coronary artery disease
- Drugs (digitalis, quinidine, amiodarone, isoproterenol) (items 14a, c)

Inverted U Wave

- LVH (item 10b)
- Severe RVH (item 10c)
- Myocardial ischemia

PP Pause > 2.0 seconds

- Sinus pause/arrest: Due to transient failure of impulse formation at the SA node; sinus rhythm resumes at a PP interval that is <u>not</u> a multiple of the basic sinus PP interval
- Sinus arrhythmia (item 2b): Phasic gradual change in PP interval
- Second-degree sinoatrial exit block, Mobitz I (Wenckebach) (item 2f): Progressive shortening of PP interval until a P wave fails to appear
- Second-degree sinoatrial exit block, Mobitz II (item 2f): Pause

followed by resumption of sinus rhythm at a PP interval that is a multiple (e.g., 2x, 3x, etc.) of the basic sinus rhythm

- Third-degree sinoatrial exit block (item 2f): Complete failure of sinuatrial conduction; cannot be differentiated from complete sinus arrest on surface ECG
- Abrupt change in autonomic tone
- "Pseudo" sinus pause due to nonconducted APCs (item 2j): P wave appears to be absent but is actually buried in the T wave — look for subtle deformity of the T wave just preceding the pause to detect nonconducted APCs

Group Beating

- Mobitz Type I second-degree AV block (item 6b)
- Blocked APCs (item 2j)
- Type II second-degree AV block (item 6c)
- Concealed His-bundle depolarizations

* * * * *

ECG CRITERIA

General Features

1a. Normal ECG

- No abnormalities of rate, rhythm, axis or P-QRS-T:

P Wave

Duration:	0.08 - 0.11 seconds
Axis:	$0 - 75^0$
Morphology:	Upright in I, II; upright or inverted in aVF; inverted or biphasic in III, aVL, V_1, V_2; small notching may be present
Amplitude:	Limb leads: < 2.5 mm; V_1: positive deflection < 1.5 mm and negative deflection < 1 mm

PR Interval

Duration:	0.12 - 0.20 seconds
PR segment:	Usually isoelectric; may be displaced in a direction opposite to the P wave; elevation usually < 0.5 mm; depression usu. < 0.8 mm

QRS Complex

Duration:	0.06 - 0.10 seconds
Axis:	-30^0 to 105^0
*Transition zone:**	V_2 - V_4
Q wave:	Small Q waves (duration < 0.04 seconds and amplitude < 2 mm) are common in most leads except aVR, V_1 and V_2
*OID:***	Right precordial leads < 0.035 seconds; left precordial leads < 0.045 seconds

---

*   Precordial leads with equal positive and negative deflection
**   Onset of intrinsicoid deflection: Beginning of QRS to peak of R wave

1a

ST Segment

Usually isoelectric; may vary from 0.5 mm below to 1 mm above baseline in limb leads; up to 3 mm concave upward elevation in precordial leads may be seen (early repolarization, item 12a)

T Wave

Morphology: Upright in I, II, V_3-V_6; inverted in aVR, V_1; may be upright, flat or biphasic in III, aVL, aVF, V_1,V_2; T wave inversion may be present in V_1-V_3 in healthy young adults (juvenile T waves, item 12b)

Amplitude: Usually < 6 mm in limb leads and < 10 mm in precordial leads

QT Interval

Corrected QT* = 0.30 - 0.46 seconds; varies inversely with heart rate

U Wave

Morphology: Upright in all leads except aVR

Amplitude: 5-25% the height of the T wave (usually < 1.5 mm)

---

* QT interval divided by the square root of the RR interval

1b. Borderline normal ECG or normal variant

- Early repolarization (item 12a)
- Juvenile T waves (item 12b)
- S wave in leads I, II, and III ($S_1 S_2 S_3$ pattern)

  Note: Present in up to 20% of healthy adults.

- RSR' or rSr' in lead V_1 with QRS duration < 0.10 seconds, r wave amplitude < 7 mm, and r' amplitude smaller than r or S waves

  Note: Seen in 2% of normals, but can also be seen in:
    ‣ RVH
    ‣ Posterior MI
    ‣ Skeletal deformities (pectus excavatum, straight back syndrome)
    ‣ High electrode placement of V_1 (in 3rd intercostal space instead of 4th)

- Tall P waves
- Notched P waves of normal duration

Note: Hyperventilation may cause prolonged PR, sinus tachycardia, and ST depression ± T wave inversion (usually seen in inferior leads).

Note: Large food intake may cause ST depression and/or T wave inversion, especially after a high carbohydrate meal.

1c

1c. Incorrect electrode placement

Limb lead reversal:

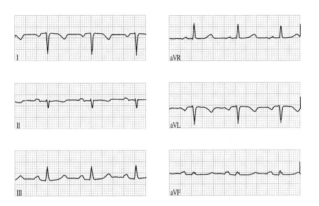

- Reversal of right and left arm leads
  - Resultant ECG mimics dextrocardia in limb leads with inversion of the P-QRS-T in leads I and aVL
  - Leads II and III transposed
  - Leads aVR and aVL transposed

  Note: To distinguish between these conditions, look at precordial leads: dextrocardia shows reverse R wave progression, while limb lead reversal shows normal R wave progression.

- Reversal of left arm and left leg leads
  - Leads I and II transposed

- ▸ Leads aVF and aVL transposed
- ▸ Lead III inverted
- • <u>Reversal of right arm and left leg leads</u>
  - ▸ Leads I, II, and III inverted
  - ▸ Leads aVR and aVF transposed

Precordial lead reversal: Typically manifests as an unexplained decrease in R wave voltage in two consecutive leads (e.g., V_1, V_2) with a return to normal R wave progression on the following leads

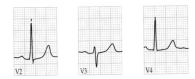

1d. Artifact

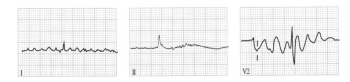

- • **AC electrical interference** (60 cycles per seconds): Due to an unstable or dry electrode, poor grounding of the ECG machine, or excessive current leak from an ECG machine too close to other electronic equipment. Rapid sine-wave changes make assessment of P waves and ST segment shifts unreliable.

1d-2a

- **Wandering baseline:** Due to an unstable electrode, deep respirations, or uncooperative patient. Evaluation of P waves, QRS voltage, and ST segment shifts are unreliable.
- **Skeletal muscle fasciculations** (e.g., shivering)
- Commonly due to **tremor** (most prominent in limb leads)
  - ▸ Parkinson's tremor simulates atrial flutter with a rate of ~ 300 per minute (4-6 cycles per second)
  - ▸ Physiologic tremor rate is 500 per minute (7-9 per second)
- **Poor standardization:** 1 mV signal is not recorded, underdamped, or overdamped; ECG recorded at half-standard or double-standard. Voltages may be inaccurate.
- **ECG recorded at double-speed or half-speed**
- **Rapid arm motion** or lead movement (e.g., teethbrushing): Can simulate VPC's or ventricular tachycardia. Commonly fools telemetry technicians and sets off monitor alarms.
- **Cautery:** Pronounced baseline interference
- **IV infusion pump:** May give appearance of rapid P waves

Atrial Rhythms

2a. Sinus rhythm

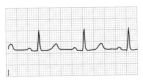

- Normal P wave axis and morphology (item 1a)
- Atrial rate is 60-100 per minute and regular (PP interval varies by < 0.16 seconds or < 10%)

2b. Sinus arrhythmia

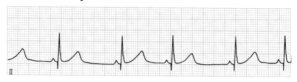

- Normal P wave morphology and axis (item 1a)
- Gradual phasic change in PP interval (may sometimes be abrupt)
- Longest and shortest PP intervals vary by >0.16 seconds or 10%

Note: Sinus arrhythmia differs from "ventriculophasic" sinus arrhythmia (which occurs in the setting of partial or complete heart block; item 5e).

2c. Sinus bradycardia

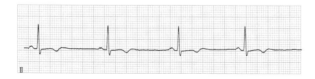

- Normal P wave axis and morphology (item 1a)
- Rate < 60 per minute

Note: If the atrial rate is < 40 per minute, think of 2:1 sinoatrial exit block (item 2f)

Note: Causes include:

- High vagal tone (normals, especially during sleep; trained athletes; Bezold-Jarisch reflex; inferior MI, pulmonary embolism)
- Myocardial infarction (usually inferior)
- Drugs (β-adrenergic blockers, verapamil, diltiazem, digitalis, Type IA, IB, IC antiarrhythmics, amiodarone, sotalol, clonidine, α-methyldopa, reserpine, guanethidine, cimetidine, lithium)
- Hypothyroidism
- Hypothermia
- Obstructive jaundice
- Hyperkalemia
- Increased intracranial pressure
- Sick sinus syndrome

2d. Sinus tachycardia

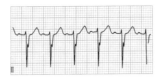

- Normal P wave axis and morphology (item 1a)
- Rate > 100 per minute

<u>Note:</u> P wave amplitude often increases and PR interval often shortens with increasing heart rate (e.g., during exercise)

<u>Note:</u> Causes include:

  ‣ Physiologic response to stress (exercise, anxiety, pain, fever, hypovolemia, hypotension, anemia)
  ‣ Thyrotoxicosis
  ‣ Myocardial ischemia/infarction
  ‣ CHF
  ‣ Myocarditis
  ‣ Pulmonary embolism
  ‣ Pheochromocytoma
  ‣ AV fistula
  ‣ Drugs (caffeine, alcohol, nicotine, cocaine, amphetamines, endogenous catecholamines, hydralazine, exogenous thyroid, atropine, aminophylline)

2e. Sinus pause or arrest

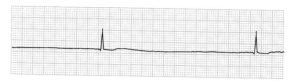

- PP interval (pause) greater than 1.6-2.0 seconds
- Sinus pause is <u>not</u> a multiple of the basic sinus PP interval

  Note: If sinus pause is a multiple of the basic PP interval, consider sinoatrial exit block (item 2f).

Note: Sinus pauses must be differentiated from:

- <u>Sinus arrhythmia</u> (item 2b): Phasic, gradual change in PP interval
- <u>Second-degree sinoatrial block, Mobitz I</u> (Wenckebach) (item 2f): Progressive shortening of PP interval until a P wave fails to appear
- <u>Second-degree sinoatrial block, Mobitz II</u> (item 2f): Sinus pause is a multiple (e.g., 2x, 3x, etc.) of the basic sinus rhythm (PP interval)
- <u>Abrupt change in autonomic tone</u>
- <u>"Pseudo" sinus pause</u> due to nonconducted atrial premature complexes (APC; item 2j): P wave appears to be absent but is actually buried in the T wave — look for subtle deformity of the T wave just preceding the pause to detect nonconducted APCs

Note: Complete failure of sinoatrial conduction (third-degree sinoatrial block; item 2f) cannot be differentiated from complete sinus arrest on surface ECG

Note: Sinus pause/arrest is due to transient failure of impulse formation at the SA node. Etiology is the same as SA exit block (item 2f).

2f. Sinoatrial (SA) block

- **FIRST-DEGREE:** Conduction of sinus impulses to the atrium is delayed, but 1:1 response is maintained; not detectable on surface ECG

- **SECOND-DEGREE:** Some sinus impulses fail to capture the atria, resulting in the intermittent absence of a P wave. Often a component of the Sick Sinus Syndrome (item 14v)

  ▸ Type I (Mobitz I):

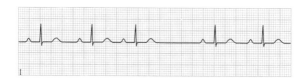

- P wave morphology and axis consistent with a sinus node origin
- "Group beating" with:

  (1) Shortening of PP interval up to pause

  (2) Constant PR interval

  (3) PP pause less than twice the normal PP interval

  ▸ Type II (Mobitz II)

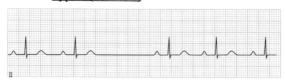

- Constant PP interval followed by a pause that is a multiple (e.g., 2x, 3x, etc.) of the normal PP interval
- The pause may be slightly less than twice the normal PP interval (usually within 0.10 seconds).

Note: Causes include:

  ▸ Drugs (digitalis, quinidine, flecainide, propafenone, procainamide)
  ▸ Hyperkalemia
  ▸ Sinus node dysfunction
  ▸ Organic heart disease
  ▸ MI
  ▸ Vagal stimulation

- **THIRD-DEGREE:** Complete failure of sinoatrial conduction; cannot be differentiated from complete sinus arrest (item 2e)

2g. Ectopic atrial rhythm

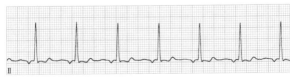

- P wave axis or morphology different from sinus node (item 1a). P waves can be upright (when atrial activity originates near the sinus node) or inverted (when the ectopic focus originates in the lower atrium).
- Atrial rate < 100 per minute

- PR interval > 0.11 seconds, and can be prolonged, normal, or short, depending on the proximity of the ectopic atrial impulse to the AV node, and whether delay is present in the AV conduction system

- QRS duration and QT interval any be normal or prolonged

Note: Inverted P waves in II, III, aVF suggest either an AV junctional rhythm with retrograde atrial activation or a low atrial rhythm. To distinguish between these mechanisms, measure the PR interval:

    ▸ PR > 0.11 seconds suggests a low atrial rhythm

    ▸ PR ≤ 0.11 seconds suggests an AV junctional rhythm

2h. Wandering atrial pacemaker

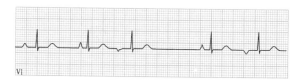

V1

- P waves with ≥ 3 morphologies (each originating from a separate atrial focus)

- Atrial rate < 100 per minute

- Varying PP and PR intervals (but may be relatively constant if atrial foci are in close proximity to each other)

- P waves may be blocked (i.e., not followed by a QRS complex), or may be conducted with a narrow or wide QRS complex.

2h-2i

<u>Note:</u> May be confused with:

- <u>Sinus rhythm with multifocal APCs</u>: Sinus rhythm with multifocal APCs demonstrates one dominant atrial pacemaker (i.e., the sinus node); in wandering atrial pacemaker, *no* dominant atrial pacemaker (i.e., no dominant P wave morphology) is present.

- <u>Atrial fibrillation/flutter</u> with a moderate ventricular response: In atrial fib/flutter, there is lack of an isoelectric baseline; in wandering atrial pacemaker, a distinct isoelectric baseline is present.

<u>Note:</u> Can be seen in normals, athletes, organic heart disease.

2i. Atrial premature complexes, normally conducted

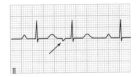

- P wave that is abnormal in configuration and premature relative to the normal PP interval
- QRS complex is similar in morphology to the QRS complex present during sinus rhythm
- The PR interval may be normal, increased, or decreased.
- The post-extrasystolic pause is usually *noncompensatory* (i.e., premature P to subsequent P wave interval is less than two PP intervals). However, an interpolated APC or a compensatory pause may be evident when sinoatrial (SA) "entrance block" is present and the SA node is not reset.

Note: Can be seen in normals, fatigue, stress, smoking, drugs (including caffeine and alcohol), organic heart disease, cor pulmonale

2j. Atrial premature complexes, nonconducted

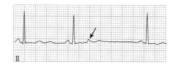

- Premature P wave with abnormal morphology that is not followed by a QRS-T complex

Note: P waves are often hidden in the preceding T wave — when you see an RR pause, look for a deformed T wave immediately preceding the pause to identify the presence of a nonconducted atrial premature beat.

Note: The sinus node is usually reset, resulting in a noncompensatory pause (item 2i)

2k. APC with aberrant conduction

- P wave occurs very early relative to the normal PP interval (also see item 2i)

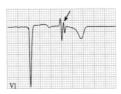

2k-2n

- Variable widening or distortion of the normal QRS (usually > 0.12 seconds). The initial QRS vector is in the same direction as the normally conducted beats, while the more terminal portion of the QRS may be in a different vector.
- QRS morphology is most often RBBB pattern, but can manifest as LBBB pattern or variable widening/distortion of the QRS. The longer refractory period of the right bundle (compared to the left bundle) increases the likelihood that an APC will conduct down the left bundle while the right bundle is still refractory.

2l. Atrial tachycardia (regular, 1:1 conduction)

- See item 2u

2m. Atrial tachycardia, repetitive (short paroxysm)

- Recurring short runs of atrial tachycardia (item 2l) interrupted by normal sinus rhythm

2n. Atrial tachycardia, multifocal

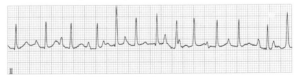

- Atrial rate >100 per minute
- P waves with ≥ 3 morphologies (each originating from a separate atrial focus)
- Varying PP and PR intervals

- P waves may be blocked (i.e., not followed by a QRS complex), or may be conducted with a narrow or aberrant QRS complex.

Note: Multifocal atrial tachycardia may be confused with:

- Sinus tachycardia with multifocal APCs, which demonstrates one dominant atrial pacemaker (i.e., the sinus node). In contrast, in multifocal atrial tachycardia, *no* dominant atrial pacemaker (i.e., no dominant P wave morphology) is present.

- Atrial fibrillation/flutter, in which there is lack of an isoelectric baseline. In contrast, multifocal atrial tachycardia demonstrates a distinct isoelectric baseline and P waves.

Note: Usually associated with some form of lung disease. Etiologies include:

- COPD

- Cor pulmonale

- Aminophylline therapy

- Hypoxia

- Organic heart disease

- CHF

- Post-op

- Sepsis

- Pulmonary edema

2o-2p

2o. Atrial tachycardia with AV block

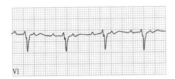

- P wave axis or morphology different from normal P waves (i.e., those arising from the sinus node; item 1a)
- Regular atrial rate at 150-240 bpm (may be as low as 100 bpm)
- Isoelectric intervals between P waves in all leads
- AV block may be second- (Mobitz I or II) or third-degree
- Atrial rhythm is regular (but may see ventriculophasic arrhythmia [item 5e])

Note: May be confused with atrial flutter. Atrial tachycardia with AV block has a distinct isoelectric baseline between P waves; atrial flutter does not, except occasionally in lead V_1.

Note: Secondary to digoxin toxicity (item 14b) in 75% and organic heart disease in 25%.

2p. Supraventricular tachycardia, unspecified

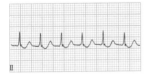

Without aberrancy

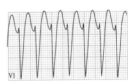

With aberrancy

- Regular rhythm
- Rate >100 per minute
- P waves not easily identified
- QRS complex is usually narrow (but occasionally aberrant)

Note: If rate is approximately 150 per minute, atrial flutter with 2:1 block may be present. Look for flutter waves in inferior leads (II, III, aVF) or V_1, or for deep inverted P waves in lead II; every other flutter wave may be buried in the QRS complex or ST segment.

2q. AV nodal reentrant tachycardia

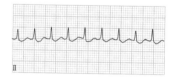

- Narrow complex SVT
- Rate of 150-250 bpm (usually 180-220 bpm)
- P wave usually buried in QRS complex or immediately follows the QRS with a short RP interval (< 0.09 sec)
- Initiates and terminates suddenly

Note: Reentry occurs in the AV node, with antegrade conduction down the slow (α) AV nodal pathway and retrograde conduction up the fast (β) AV nodal pathway. Often initiated by APCs. Accounts for 60-70% of SVTs. Carotid sinus massage slows and frequently terminates tachycardia.

Note: Occurs commonly in normals.

2r-2s

2r. Atypical AV nodal re-entrant tachycardia

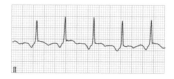

- Narrow complex SVT with long RP interval (i.e., RP > ½ PP interval)
- P waves usually negative in II III, and aVF

Note: ECG indistinguishable from atrial tachycardia.

Note: Reentry circuit in AV node with antegrade conduction down the rapid (β) AV node pathway and retrograde conduction up the slow (α) pathway. May require an EP study to diagnose. Found in 5-10% of patients with AV node reentry (i.e., 2-5% of SVTs). Carotid sinus massage may terminate the tachycardia.

2s. AV reentrant tachycardia (WPW syndrome); orthodromic SVT

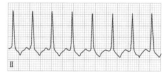

- Regular rhythm
- Rate 150-250 bpm
- Usually a short RP SVT (but may have a long RP interval if there is slow retrograde [VA] conduction)

- Sudden initiation and termination

Note: SVT often initiated by APCs. Terminates suddenly with carotid sinus massage.

Note: Associated with Wolff-Parkinson-White syndrome and concealed bypass tracts. The hearts are usually normal in these conditions but can be associated with Ebstein's anomaly, cardiomyopathy, or mitral valve prolapse.

2t. Orthodromic SVT with prolonged VA conduction

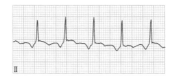

- Narrow QRS complex SVT with a long RP interval
- P waves are usually negative in II, III, aVF

Note: ECG is indistinguishable from atrial tachycardia.

Note: Represents an orthodromic SVT involving a bypass tract (usually posterior) with slow retrograde conduction. Often an incessant (continuous, longstanding) tachycardia. May be difficult to distinguish from automatic atrial and intraatrial re-entrant tachycardias (item 2u), and require an EP study to diagnose. Carotid sinus massage may terminates the tachycardia.

2u. Atrial tachycardia (automatic or intra-atrial reentry)

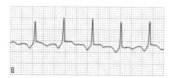

- Regular rhythm
- Atrial rate 100-200 bpm
- P wave morphology differs from sinus P wave
- Usually a long RP SVT but may have a short RP interval (i.e., < 50% of PP interval) if first-degree AV block is present

<u>Note:</u> May be due to automatic atrial tachycardia or intraatrial reentry. Accounts for 10% of SVTs. Carotid sinus massage produces AV block but does not terminate the tachycardia.

<u>Note:</u> Nonsustained atrial tachycardia is common in normals, whereas the sustained form is more common in organic heart disease, especially MI and cor pulmonale.

2v. Sinus node reentrant tachycardia

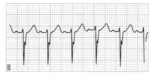

- Regular rhythm
- Sudden onset and termination

- Rate 100-160 bpm
- P waves same as sinus P waves

Note: ECG indistinguishable from sinus tachycardia

Note: Involves reentry in or around the sinus node. Accounts for 5-10% of SVTs. Carotid sinus massage produces AV block but does not terminate the tachycardia.

Note: Seen in normals, but more common in organic heart disease.

2w. Supraventricular tachycardia (paroxysmal)

- Onset and termination of SVT (item 2p) is sudden
- SVT is episodic and does not persist throughout the entire tracing

2x. Atrial flutter

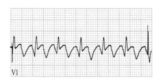

- Rapid regular atrial undulations (flutter or "F" waves) usually at a rate of 240-340 per minute

  Note: Flutter rate may be faster (> 340 per minute) in children, and slower (200-240 per minute) in the presence of antiarrhythmic drugs (Type IA, IC, III) and/or massively dilated atria.

Note: ECG artifact due to Parkinsonian tremor (~ 4-6 cycles second) can simulate flutter waves. Look for evidence of distinct superimposed P waves proceeding each QRS complex, especially in leads I, II, or V_1.

- Typical atrial flutter morphology usually present:
  - ‣ Leads II, III, AVF: Inverted F waves without an isoelectric baseline ("picket-fence" or "sawtooth" appearance)
  - ‣ Lead V_1: Small positive deflections usually with a distinct isoelectric baseline
- Atypical atrial flutter can exhibit upright F waves in inferior leads
- QRS complex may be normal or aberrant
- Rate and regularity of QRS complexes depend on the AV conduction sequence
  - ‣ AV conduction ratio (ratio of flutter waves to QRS complexes) is usually fixed and an even number (e.g., 2:1, 4:1), but may vary.

    Note: Odd-numbered conduction ratios of 1:1 and 3:1 are uncommon. Atrial flutter with 1:1 AV conduction often conducts aberrantly, resulting in a wide QRS tachycardia that may be confused with VT. In untreated patients, $\geq$ 4:1 block suggests the coexistence of AV conduction disease.

    Note: Carotid sinus massage typically causes a transient increase in AV block and slowing of the ventricular response, without a change in the atrial flutter rate. At times, no effect is seen. When atrial flutter with 2:1 AV block is suspected, carotid sinus massage may unmask flutter waves and help confirm the diagnosis. Upon discontinuation of carotid sinus massage, the usual response is return to the original ventricular rate.

▸ Complete heart block with a junctional or ventricular escape rhythm may be present.

Note: Think digitalis toxicity when complete heart block with junctional tachycardia is present.

Note: Flutter waves can deform QRS, ST and/or T to mimic intraventricular conduction delay and/or myocardial ischemia.

Note: Etiology is the same as for atrial fibrillation (item 2y).

2y. Atrial fibrillation

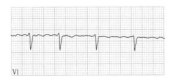

- P waves absent
- Atrial activity is totally irregular and represented by fibrillatory (f) waves of varying amplitude, duration and morphology, causing random oscillation of the baseline

  Note: Atrial activity is best seen in leads V_1, V_2, II, III, aVF.

- Ventricular rhythm is typically irregularly irregular

  Note: If the RR interval is regular, second- or third-degree AV block (item 6e) is present.

  Note: Digoxin toxicity may result in regularization of the QRS due to complete heart block with junctional tachycardia.

- Ventricular rate is usually 100-180 per minute in the absence of drugs

  <u>Note:</u> If the rate without AV blocking drugs is less than 100 beats per minute, AV conduction system disease is likely to be present.

  <u>Note:</u> Consider Wolff-Parkinson-White Syndrome (item 6h) if the ventricular rate is > 200 per minute and the QRS is > 0.12 seconds. The 12-lead ECG during sinus rhythm should show a short PR interval and a wide QRS complex with initial slurring (delta wave).

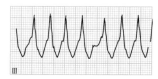

  <u>Note:</u> Conditions mimicking atrial fibrillation include:
  - ▸ Multifocal atrial tachycardia (item 2n)
  - ▸ Paroxysmal atrial tachycardia with block (item 2o)
  - ▸ Atrial flutter (item 2r)

  <u>Note:</u> Etiologies include:

- ▸ Mitral valve disease

- ▸ Organic heart disease

- ▸ Hypertension

- ▸ Post-CABG

- MI
- Thyrotoxicosis
- Pulmonary embolism
- Post-operative state
- Hypoxia
- COPD
- Atrial septal defect
- WPW
- Sick Sinus Syndrome
- Alcohol
- Normals

2z. Retrograde atrial activation

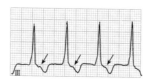

- Inverted P waves in leads II, III and aVF

Note: Look for retrograde P waves after ventricular premature complexes and other junctional, ventricular, or low ectopic atrial rhythms.

AV Junctional Rhythms

3a. AV junctional premature complexes

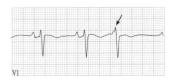

- Premature QRS complex (relative to the basic RR interval), which may be narrow or aberrant

- The P wave may precede the QRS by ≤ 0.11 seconds (retrograde atrial activation, item 2t), may be buried in the QRS (and not visualized), or may follow the QRS complex

- Inverted P waves in leads II, III, aVF (item 2t) and upright P waves in leads I and aVL are commonly seen due to the spread of atrial activation from near the AV node and in a superior and leftward direction (i.e., away from the inferior leads and toward the left lateral leads).

  Note: The atrium may occasionally be activated by the sinus node, resulting in a normal sinus P wave. This occurs when retrograde block exists between the AV junctional focus and the atrium, or the sinus node activates the atrium before the AV junctional impulse.

  Note: A constant coupling interval and noncompensatory pause are usually present.

  Note: Seen in normals and organic heart disease.

3b. AV junctional escape complexes

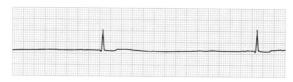

- Typically narrow QRS complex beat(s) that follow the previous conducted beat at a coupling interval corresponding to a rate of 40-60 per minute
- P wave may precede (PR < 0.11 seconds), be buried in, or follow the QRS complex (similar to AV junctional premature beats; item 3a)
- QRS morphology is similar to the sinus or supraventricular impulse

<u>Note:</u> QRS complex occurs as a secondary phenomenon in response to decreased sinus impulse formation or conduction, high-degree AV block, or after a pause following termination of atrial tachycardia, atrial flutter, or atrial fibrillation.

3c. AV junctional rhythm, accelerated

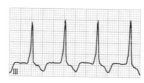

- Regular QRS rhythm at rate >60 per minute

- P wave may proceed, be buried in, or follow the QRS complex
- QRS is usually narrow but may be wide if aberrant or preexisting IVCD
- Relationship between atrial and ventricular rates may vary:
  - If retrograde (VA) block is present, the atria remain in sinus rhythm and *AV dissociation* (item 5d) will be present
  - If retrograde atrial activation (item 2t) occurs, a constant QRS-P interval is usually present (occasionally there is 2:1 VA conduction)

Note: Think digitalis toxicity (item 14b) if atrial fibrillation or flutter with a regular RR is seen — this often represents complete heart block with accelerated junctional rhythm.

Note: Can be seen in acute myocardial infarction (usually inferior), myocarditis, digitalis toxicity, and following open heart surgery.

3d. AV junctional rhythm

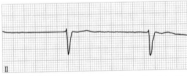

- P wave and QRS complex as described in item 3a
- RR interval of escape rhythm is usually constant (< 0.04 seconds variation)
- Usual heart rate is between 40-60 BPM

Note: Often associated with isorhythmic AV dissociation (item 5d) and retrograde atrial activation (item 2t).

Ventricular Rhythms

4a. VPCs, uniform, fixed coupling

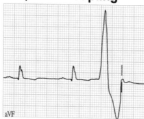

Requires all of the following:

- A wide, notched or slurred QRS complex that is:

    ▸ Premature relative to the normal RR interval, *and*

    ▸ Not preceded by a P wave (except when late coupled VPCs follow a sinus P wave; in this case, the PR interval is usually ≤ 0.11 seconds)

Note: QRS is almost always > 0.12 seconds, but VPCs originating high in the interventricular septum may have a relatively normal QRS duration.

Note: When a VPC occurs just distal to the site of bundle branch block and near the interventricular septum, the QRS of the VPC may be narrower than the QRS of the bundle branch block.

Note: Initial direction of the QRS is often different from the QRS during sinus rhythm.

- Secondary ST & T wave changes in a direction opposite to the major deflection of the QRS (i.e., ST depression & T wave inversion in leads with a dominant R wave; ST elevation and upright T wave in leads with a dominant S wave or QS complex)
- Coupling interval (relation of VPCs to the preceding QRS) is constant (or varies by < 0.08 seconds)
- Morphology of VPCs in any given lead is the same (i.e., uniform)

Note: Retrograde capture of atria may occur (item 2t)

Note: A full compensatory pause (PP interval containing the VPC is twice the normal PP interval) is usually evident, but this relationship may be altered if sinus arrhythmia is also present. A partial compensatory pause may follow a VPC when ventriculoatrial conduction penetrates and resets the sinus node. Less commonly, interpolated VPCs occur, manifesting as VPCs that are interposed between two consecutive sinus beats without disrupting the basic sinus rhythm; interpolated VPCs result in neither a partial nor a full compensatory pause.

Note: Clues on the electrocardiogram suggestive of a ventricular (rather than atrial) origin of an ectopic beat include an initial QRS vector different from the sinus beats, QRS duration > 0.12 seconds, retrograde P waves (caused by retrograde conduction through the AV node), and the presence of a full compensatory pause.

Note: Seen in normals and all causes of ventricular tachycardia (item 4f).

4b. VPCs, nonfixed coupling

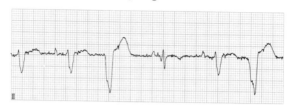

- Relationship of VPCs to preceding QRS (coupling interval) is variable
- See item 4a for QRS morphology

Note: This should raise the suspicion of parasystole (item 4e)

4c. VPCs, multiform

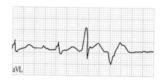

- VPCs with ≥ 2 morphologies
- Fixed or nonfixed coupling may be present

Note: Although multiform VPCs are usually multifocal in origin (i.e., originate from more than one ventricular focus), a single ventricular focus can produce VPCs of varying morphology.

4d-4e

4d. VPCs, in pairs (two consecutive)

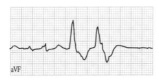

- Two consecutive ventricular premature complexes (items 4a, c) of not necessarily the same morphology

4e. Ventricular parasystole

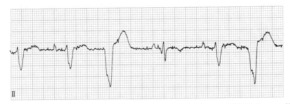

- Frequent ventricular premature complexes (VPCs) usually at a rate of 30-50 per minute with the interectopic intervals a multiple (2x, 3x, etc.) of the shortest interectopic interval present (since the parasystolic focus fires at a regular rate and inscribes a QRS complex whenever the ventricles are not refractory)
- Resultant VPCs vary in relationship to the preceding sinus or supraventricular beats (i.e., nonfixed coupling)
- VPCs typically manifest the same morphology (which resembles a VPC, item 4a) unless fusion occurs (item 5a)

Note: Fusion complexes, resulting from simultaneous activation of the ventricles by atrial and parasystolic impulses, are commonly seen but are not required for the diagnosis.

Note: Exit block from a parasystolic focus may occur and result in absence of a ventricular ectopic beat when it would be expected to occur.

Note: Ventricular parasystole is due to the presence of an ectopic ventricular focus that activates the ventricles independent of the basic sinus or supraventricular rhythm, and is protected from depolarization by an entrance block. The ventricular focus fires at a regular cycle length and results in a VPC that bears no constant relationship (nonfixed coupling) to the previous sinus beat. In contrast to ventricular parasystole, uniform VPC's due to local reentry initiated by prior sinus activation of the ventricle show fixed coupling.

Note: Think of parasystole when you see ventricular premature complexes with nonfixed coupling and fusion beats.

4f. Ventricular tachycardia

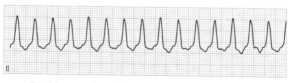

- Rapid succession of three or more premature ventricular beats (item 4a) at a rate > 100 per minute

4f

- RR interval is usually regular but may be irregular
- Abrupt onset and termination of arrhythmia is evident
- AV dissociation (item 5d) is common
- On occasion, retrograde atrial activation (item 2t) and capture occur

Note: Ventriculoatrial conduction may occur at 1:1, or may manifest variable, fixed, or complete block; ventriculoatrial Wenckebach may also occur.

Note: In the setting of a wide QRS tachycardia, certain findings may help distinguish ventricular tachycardia from supraventricular tachycardia with aberrancy (Figure 1).

Note: Rarely, VT can present as a narrow QRS complex tachycardia.

Note: Bidirectional VT is a rare type of VT in which the QRS complexes in any given lead alternate in polarity. It is most often caused by digitalis toxicity.

Note: Seen in:

- Organic heart disease
- Hypokalemia
- Hyperkalemia
- Hypoxia
- Acidosis
- Drugs (digitalis toxicity, antirrhythmics, phenothiazines, tricyclics, caffeine, alcohol, nicotine)
- Mitral valve prolapse
- Occasionally in normals

4f

Figure 1. Differentiation of Wide QRS Tachycardia

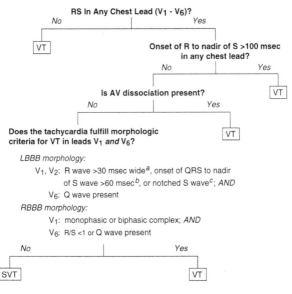

RS In Any Chest Lead (V₁ - V₆)?

No → VT

Yes → **Onset of R to nadir of S >100 msec in any chest lead?**

No → **Is AV dissociation present?**

Yes → VT

No → **Does the tachycardia fulfill morphologic criteria for VT in leads V₁ *and* V₆?**

Yes → VT

LBBB morphology:

V₁, V₂: R wave >30 msec wide[a], onset of QRS to nadir of S wave >60 msec[b], or notched S wave[c]; *AND*

V₆: Q wave present

RBBB morphology:

V₁: monophasic or biphasic complex; *AND*

V₆: R/S <1 or Q wave present

No → SVT

Yes → VT

VT = Ventricular tachycardia
SVT = Supraventricular tachycardia

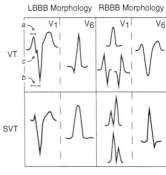

LBBB Morphology   RBBB Morphology

Circulation 1991; 83:1649

4g

4g. Accelerated idioventricular rhythm

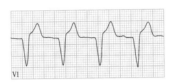

- Regular or slightly irregular ventricular (i.e., wide complex) rhythm
- Rate of 60-110 per minute
- QRS morphology similar to VPCs (item 4a)
- AV dissociation (item 5d), ventricular capture complexes (item 5c), and fusion beats (item 5a) are common because of the competition between the normal sinus and ectopic ventricular rhythms.

Note: Unlike ventricular tachycardia, AIVR is not associated with an adverse prognosis.

Note: Seen in:

▶ Myocardial ischemia

▶ Following coronary reperfusion

▶ Digitalis toxicity

▶ Occasionally in normals

4h. Ventricular escape beats or rhythm

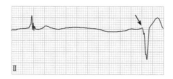

- Regular or slightly irregular ventricular rhythm
- Rate of 30-40 per minute (can be 20-50 per min)
- QRS morphology similar to VPCs (item 4a)

Note: QRS complex occurs as a secondary phenomenon in response to decreased sinus impulse formation or conduction, high-degree AV block, or after the pause following termination of atrial tachycardia, atrial flutter, or atrial fibrillation.

4i. Ventricular fibrillation

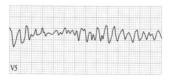

- An extremely rapid and irregular ventricular rhythm demonstrating:
  - ▸ Chaotic and irregular deflections of varying amplitude and contour
  - ▸ Absence of distinct P waves, QRS complexes, and T waves

4j-5a

4j. Torsade de Pointes

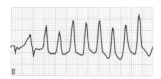

- Polymorphic wide complex ventricular tachycardia (cycles of 3 or more beats with alternating polarity in a sinusoidal pattern) occurring in the setting of a prolonged QT interval.

  Note: Occurs in paroxysms but can degenerate into ventricular fibrillation.

  Note: Often preceded by long-short R-R cycles.

  Note: VT of similar morphology in the absence of QT prolongation is called polymorphic VT.

AV Interactions

5a. Fusion complexes

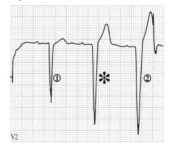

- Simultaneous activation of the ventricle from two sources, resulting in a QRS complex intermediate in morphology between the QRS complexes of each source

Note: Fusion complexes may be seen with:

- ▸ Ventricular premature complexes (item 4a-d)
- ▸ Ventricular tachycardia (item 4f)
- ▸ Ventricular parasystole (item 4e)
- ▸ Accelerated idioventricular rhythm (item 4g)
- ▸ Wolff-Parkinson-White Syndrome (item 6h)
- ▸ Paced rhythm

5b. Reciprocal (echo) complexes

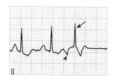

- An impulse activates a chamber (atria or ventricle), returns to site of origin, and reactivates the same chamber again
- A form of nonsustained reentry

5c. Ventricular capture complexes

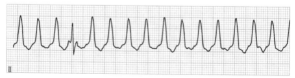

5c-5d

- Occurs when an atrial impulse is conducted to and stimulates the ventricles during ventricular tachycardia. The "captured" ventricle results in a QRS complex similar to that during sinus rhythm

Note: The presence of a ventricular capture complex in the setting of a wide QRS tachycardia strongly suggests the diagnosis of ventricular tachycardia.

5d. AV dissociation

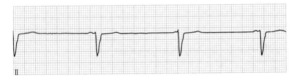

- Atrial and ventricular rhythms are independent of each other
- Ventricular rate is equal to or faster than the atrial rate

Note: AV dissociation is a secondary phenomenon resulting from some other disturbance of cardiac rhythm. Examples include:

- AV dissociation may involve:
  - A ventricular rate that is faster than the normal atrial rate because of acceleration of a subsidiary pacemaker (e.g., junctional or ventricular tachycardia, myocardial ischemia, digitalis toxicity, post-operative state)
  - A ventricular rate that is faster than the normal atrial rate because of slowing of the atrial rate (sinus bradycardia, sinus arrest, sinoatrial exit block, high vagal tone, post-cardioversion, β-blockers) below the intrinsic rate of a subsidiary AV junctional or ventricular pacemaker

> ▸ A ventricular rate that is slower than the atrial rate because of AV block

5e. Ventriculophasic sinus arrhythmia

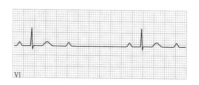

- PP interval containing a QRS complex is shorter than the PP interval without a QRS complex

<u>Note:</u> Occurs in 30-50% with partial or complete AV block.

AV Conduction Abnormalities

6a. AV block, 1°

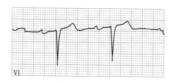

- PR interval ≥ 0.20 seconds (usually 0.21-0.40 seconds but may be as long as 0.80 seconds)
- Each P wave is followed by a QRS complex

6a-6b

Note: The PR interval represents the time from the onset of atrial depolarization to the onset of ventricular repolarization (i.e., conduction time from the atrium → AV node → His bundle → Purkinje system → ventricles). It does not reflect conduction from the sinus node to the atrial tissue. Therefore, a prolonged PR interval with a narrow QRS complex identifies the site of block in the AV node. If the QRS is wide, conduction delay or block typically occurs in the His-Purkinje system (although block in the AV node can manifest as a prolonged PR and wide QRS if bundle branch block or rate-dependant aberrancy is present).

Note: Etiologies include:

- ▸ Normals
- ▸ Athletes
- ▸ High vagal tone
- ▸ Drugs (digitalis, quinidine, procainamide, flecainide, propafenone, amiodarone, sotalol propranolol, verapamil)
- ▸ Acute rheumatic fever
- ▸ Myocarditis
- ▸ Congenital heart disease (atrial septal defect, patent ductus arteriosus)

6b. AV block, 2° - Mobitz Type I (Wenckebach)

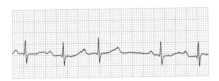

- Progressive prolongation of the PR interval and progressive shortening of the RR interval until a P wave is blocked

  Note: The progressive shortening of the RR interval is due to a decrease in the increment of PR interval prolongation.

- RR interval containing the nonconducted P wave is less than two PP intervals

Note: Classical Wenckebach periodicity may not always be evident, especially when sinus arrhythmia is present or an abrupt change in autonomic tone occurs.

Note: In Type I block with high conduction ratios (i.e., infrequent pauses), the PR interval of the beats immediately preceding the blocked P wave may be equal to each other, suggesting Type II block. In these situations, it is best to compare the PR intervals immediately before and after the blocked P wave; differences in the PR intervals suggest Type I block, whereas a constant PR interval suggests Type II block.

Note: Mobitz Type I results in "group" or "pattern beating" due to the presence of nonconducted P waves. Other causes of group beating include:

- Blocked APCs (item 2j)
- Type II second-degree AV block (item 6c)
- Concealed His-bundle depolarizations: Premature His depolarizations render the AV node refractory to subsequent sinus beats, resulting in blocked P waves and pseudo-AV block.

Note: Type I block usually occurs at the level of the AV node, resulting in a narrow QRS complex. In contrast, Mobitz Type II block usually occurs within or below the bundle of His, and is associated with a wide QRS complex in 80% of cases.

6b-6c

<u>Note:</u> Etiologies include:

- ► Normals
- ► Athletes
- ► Drugs (digitalis, β-blocker, calcium blockers, clonidine, α-methyldopa, flecainide, sotalol, amiodarone encainide, propafenone, lithium)
- ► Myocardial infarction (especially inferior)
- ► Acute rheumatic fever
- ► Myocarditis

6c. AV block, 2° - Mobitz Type II

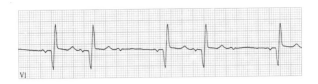

- Regular sinus or atrial rhythm (item 2g) with intermittent nonconducted P waves and no evidence for atrial prematurity
- PR interval in the conducted beats is constant
- RR interval containing the nonconducted P wave is equal to two PP intervals

<u>Note:</u> Type II second-degree AV block usually occurs within or below the bundle of His; the QRS is wide in 80% of cases.

<u>Note:</u> 2:1 AV block can be Mobitz Type I or II (Table 1).

Note: In Type I block with high conduction rates (e.g., 10:9 conduction), the PR interval of the beats immediately preceding the blocked P wave may be equal, suggesting Type II block. In these situations, it is best to compare the PR interval immediately before and after the blocked P wave; differences in the PR interval suggest Type I block, whereas a constant PR interval is evidence for Type II block, which is almost always due to organic heart disease.

Table 1. Features Suggesting the Mechanism of 2:1 AV Block

Feature	Mechanism	
	Mobitz Type I	Mobitz Type II
QRS duration	Narrow	Wide
Response to maneuvers that increase heart rate & AV conduction (e.g., atropine, exercise)	Block improves	Block worsens
Response to maneuvers that reduce heart rate & AV conduction (e.g., carotid sinus massage)	Block worsens	Block improves
Develops during acute MI	Inferior MI	Anterior MI
Other	Mobitz I on another part of ECG	History of syncope

6d-6e

6d. AV block, 2:1

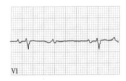

- Regular sinus or atrial rhythm with two P waves for each QRS complex (i.e., every other P wave is nonconducted)

Note: Can be Mobitz Type I or II second-degree AV block (see Table 1, previous page).

6e. AV block, 3°

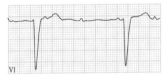

- Atrial impulses consistently fail to reach the ventricles, resulting in atrial and ventricular rhythms that are independent of each other
- PR interval varies
- PP and RR intervals are constant
- Atrial rate is usually faster than ventricular rate
- Ventricular rhythm is maintained by a junctional or idioventricular escape rhythm or a ventricular pacemaker

Note: The P wave may precede, be buried within (and not visualized), or follow the QRS to deform the ST segment or T wave.

Note: Ventriculophasic sinus arrhythmia (item 5a) may be present in 30-50%.

Note: Complete heart block may present with an atrial rate slower than the ventricular escape rate. This is identified by the presence of nonconducted P waves when the AV node and ventricle are not refractory.

Note: Causes of complete heart block include:

- **MYOCARDIAL INFARCTION:** 5-15% of acute myocardial infarctions are complicated by complete heart block: In inferior MI, complete heart block is usually preceded by first-degree AV block or Type I second-degree AV block, usually occurs at the level of the AV node, is typically transient (< 1 week), and is usually associated with a stable junctional escape rhythm (narrow QRS; rate ≥ 40 BPM). In anterior MI, complete heart block occurs as a result of extensive damage to the left ventricle, is typically preceded by Type II second-degree AV block or bifasicular block, and is associated with mortality rates as high as 70% (due to pump failure rather than heart block per se)

- **DEGENERATIVE DISEASES** of the conduction system (Lev's disease, Lenegre's disease)

- **INFILTRATIVE DISEASES** of the myocardium (e.g., amyloid, sarcoid)

- **DIGITALIS TOXICITY:** One of the most common causes of reversible complete AV block; usually associated with a junctional escape rhythm (narrow QRS), which is often accelerated

► **ENDOCARDITIS:** Inflammation and edema of the septum and peri-AV nodal tissues may cause conduction failure and complete heart block; PR prolongation usually precedes this event

► **ADVANCED HYPERKALEMIA** (death is usually from ventricular tachyarrhytmias)

► **LYME DISEASE:** Caused by a tick-borne spirochete (Borrelia burgdorferi), this disorder begins with a characteristic skin rash (erythema chronicum migrans), and may be followed in subsequent weeks to months by joint, cardiac and neurological involvement. Cardiac involvement includes AV block, which may be partial or complete, usually occurs at the level of the AV node, and may be accompanied by syncope

► **OTHERS:** Myocardial contusion, acute rheumatic fever, aortic valve disease

6f. AV block, variable

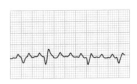

• Varying degrees of AV block (1°, 2°, 3°)

<u>Note:</u> Consider this diagnosis in atrial flutter with variable flutter-to-R wave intervals after ruling out third-degree AV block

6g. Short PR interval (with sinus rhythm and normal QRS duration)

- Normal P wave (item 1a)
- PR interval <0.12 sec
- No delta wave (QRS <0.11 sec)
- No sinus rhythm with AV dissociation

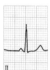

<u>Note:</u> Must be distinguished from other conditions associated with a short PR interval:

- ▸ Initial slurring (delta wave) of a wide QRS suggests WPW
- ▸ If the P waves are inverted in leads II, III, aVF, either AV junctional rhythm with retrograde atrial activation or low atrial rhythm should be considered
- ▸ Isorhythmic dissociation may appear to have sinus rhythm with a short PR interval; however on close inspection, the P waves merge in and out of (are dissociated from) the QRS complex without evidence of a short PR interval of fixed duration

6h. Wolff-Parkinson-White pattern

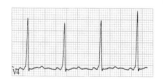

Normal sinus rhythm

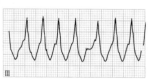

Atrial fibrillation

- Normal P wave axis and morphology (item 1a)
- PR interval < 0.12 seconds (rarely > 0.12 seconds)

  Note: AV conduction over the accessory pathway (Bundle of Kent) bypasses the AV node (and AV nodal conduction delay), resulting in pre-excitation of the ventricles and a short PR interval

- Initial slurring of the QRS (delta wave), resulting in an abnormally wide QRS (> 0.10 seconds)

  Note: The QRS duration is ≤ 0.10 seconds in 30%. In these cases, the ventricles are depolarized almost entirely by the normal AV conduction system, with minimal contribution from antegrade conduction along the accessory pathway.

  Note: The widened QRS complexes represent fusion between electrical wavefronts conducted down the accessory pathway (delta wave) and the AV node. Differing degrees of pre-excitation (fusion) may be present, resulting in variability in the delta wave and QRS duration.

- Secondary ST-T wave changes (opposite in direction to main deflection of QRS)

Note: The PJ interval (beginning of P wave to the J point (i.e., end of QRS complex) is constant and ≤ 0.26 seconds. This is due to an inverse relationship between the PR interval and QRS duration — if the PR interval shortens, the QRS widens; if the PR interval lengthens, the QRS narrows.

Note: Think WPW when atrial fibrillation or flutter is associated with a QRS that varies in width (generally wide) and has a rate >200 per minute

Note: Atrial fibrillation can conduct extremely rapidly, resulting in aberrant conduction and an irregular wide complex tachycardia, which resembles VT and can degenerate into VF.

OVERVIEW: Wolff-Parkinson-White syndrome (WPW) is characterized by the presence of an abnormal muscular network of specialized conduction tissue that connects the atrium to the ventricle and bypasses conduction through the AV node. It is found in 0.2-0.4% of the overall population and is more common in males and younger patients. Most patients with WPW do not have structural heart disease, although there is an increased prevalence of this disorder among patients with Epstein's anomaly (downward displacement of the tricuspid valve into the right ventricle due to anomalous attachment of the tricuspid leaflets), hypertrophic cardiomyopathy, mitral valve prolapse, and dilated cardiomyopathy. Two types of accessory pathways (AP) exist: In *manifest* AP, antegrade conduction occurs over the AP and results in pre-excitation on baseline ECG (which may be intermittent). In *concealed* AP, antegrade conduction occurs via the AV node and retrograde conduction occurs over the AP, so pre-excitation is not evident on the baseline ECG. Approximately 50% of patients with WPW manifest tachyarrhythmias, of which 80% is AV reentry tachycardia, 15% is atrial fibrillation, and 5% is atrial flutter. Asymptomatic individuals have an excellent prognosis. For patients with recurrent tachycardias, the overall prognosis is good but sudden death may occur. The presence of delta waves and secondary repolarization abnormalities can lead to a false positive or false negative diagnoses of ventricular hypertrophy, bundle branch block, and acute myocardial infarction. The polarity of the delta waves can be used to predict the location of the bypass tract.

Intraventricular Conduction Disturbances

7a. RBBB, incomplete

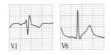

- RBBB morphology (rSR' in V_1; item 7b) with a QRS duration between 0.09 and less than 0.12 seconds

Note: Other causes of RSR' pattern < 0.12 seconds in lead V_1 include:

- ▸ Normal variant (present in ~ 2% of healthy adults) (item 1b)
- ▸ Right ventricular hypertrophy (item 10c)
- ▸ Posterior wall MI (item 11l)
- ▸ Incorrect lead placement (electrode for lead V_1 placed in 3rd instead of 4th intercostal space) (item 1c)
- ▸ Skeletal deformities (e.g., pectus excavatum)
- ▸ Atrial septal defect (items 14i, 14j)

7b. RBBB, complete

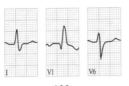

- Prolonged QRS duration (≥ 0.12 seconds)
- Secondary R wave (R') in leads V_1 and V_2 (rsR' or rSR') with R' usually taller than the initial R wave
- Delayed onset of intrinsicoid deflection (beginning of QRS to peak of R wave > 0.05 seconds) in V_1 and V_2
- Secondary ST & T-wave changes (T wave inversion; downsloping ST segment may or may not be present) in leads V_1 and V_2 (item 12g)
- Wide slurred S wave in leads I, V_5, and V_6

Note: In RBBB, mean QRS axis is determined by the initial unblocked 0.06-0.08 seconds of QRS, and should be normal unless left anterior fascicular block (item 7c) or left posterior fascicular block (item 7d) is present.

Note: RBBB does not interfere with the ECG diagnosis of ventricular hypertrophy or Q-wave MI.

Note: Can be seen in:

- Occasionally in normal adults (incidence ~ 2/1000) without underlying structural heart disease (unlike LBBB). These patients have essentially the same prognosis as the general population. However, among patients with coronary artery disease, RBBB is associated with a 2-fold increase in morality (compared to patients with coronary disease but without bundle branch block).
- Hypertensive heart disease
- Myocarditis
- Cardiomyopathy
- Rheumatic heart disease

- ▸ Cor pulmonale (acute or chronic)
- ▸ Degenerative disease of the conduction system (Lenegre's disease) or sclerosis of the cardiac skeleton (Lev's disease)
- ▸ Ebstein's anomaly

7c. Left anterior fascicular block

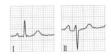

- Left axis deviation with mean QRS axis between -45° and -90° (item 9c)
- qR complex (or an R wave) in leads I and aVL
- rS complex in lead III
- Normal or slightly prolonged QRS duration (0.08-0.10 seconds)
- No other factors responsible for left axis deviation:
  - ▸ LVH (items 10a, b)
  - ▸ Inferior wall MI (items 11e, k)
  - ▸ Emphysema (chronic lung disease) (item 14m)
  - ▸ Left bundle branch block (item 7f)
  - ▸ Ostium premium atrial septal defect (item 14j)
  - ▸ Severe hyperkalemia (item 14f)

Note: LAFB may result in a false-positive diagnosis of LVH based on voltage criteria using leads I or aVL.

Note: Poor R wave progression is common.

Note: Left anterior fascicular block can mask the presence of inferior wall MI.

Note: When QS complexes are present in the inferior leads, inferior MI and LAFB may both be present.

Note: The anterior fascicle of the left bundle branch supplies the Purkinje fibers to the anterior and lateral walls of the left ventricle.

Note: Seen in organic heart disease, congenital heart disease, and rarely in normals.

7d. Left posterior fascicular block

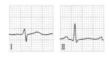

- Right axis deviation with mean QRS axis between +100° and +180° (item 9d)

- $S_1 Q_3$ pattern (deep S wave in lead I; Q wave in lead III)

- Normal or slightly prolonged QRS duration (0.08-0.10 seconds)

- No other factors responsible for right axis deviation:
  - ‣ RVH (item 10c)
  - ‣ Vertical heart
  - ‣ Emphysema (chronic lung disease) (item 14m)

7d-7e

- ▸ Pulmonary embolism (item 14n)
- ▸ Lateral wall MI (items 10d, j)
- ▸ Dextrocardia (item 14k)
- ▸ Lead reversal (item 1c)
- ▸ Wolff-Parkinson-White (item 6h)

Note: Left posterior fascicular block can mask the presence of lateral wall MI.

Note: Compared to the left anterior fascicle, the left posterior fascicle is shorter, thicker, and receives blood supply from both left and right coronary arteries. Isolated left posterior fascicular block (LPFB) is much less prevalent than left bundle branch block, right bundle branch block, or left anterior fascicular block.

Note: Coronary artery disease is the most common cause of LPFB; when it develops during acute MI, multivessel coronary disease and extensive infarction are usually present, and the prognosis is poor. LPFB is rarely seen in normals.

7e. LBBB, with ST-T waves suggestive of acute myocardial injury or infarction

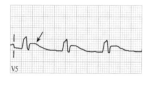 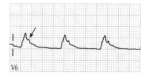

- Fulfills criteria for LBBB (item 7f) (also valid for LBBB due to artificial pacemaker)

- Three criteria with independent value for diagnosing acute myocardial injury in setting of LBBB (in descending order of significance):
    - ST elevation ≥ 1 mm concordant to (same direction as) the major deflection of the QRS
    - ST depression ≥ 1 mm in V_1, V_2, or V_3
    - ST elevation ≥ 5 mm discordant with (opposite direction to) the major deflection of the QRS

<u>Note:</u> In the setting of LBBB, acute myocardial infarction is very difficult to diagnosis and the usual criteria do not apply. Q waves are often normally present in the anteroseptal leads with LBBB and cannot be considered pathologic. In addition, ST depression and T wave inversion are commonly seen in the absence of acute ischemia.

<u>Note:</u> VPCs showing QR or QRS (but not QS) complexes during suspected MI lend further support for this diagnosis.

7f. LBBB, complete

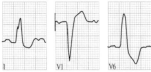

- Prolonged QRS duration (≥ 0.12 seconds)
- Delayed onset of intrinsicoid deflection (i.e., beginning of QRS to peak of R wave > 0.05 seconds) in leads I, V_5, V_6
- Broad monophasic R waves in leads I, V_5, V_6 that are usually notched or slurred

7f-7h

- Secondary ST & T wave changes opposite in direction to the major QRS deflection (i.e., ST depression & T wave inversion in leads I, V_5, V_6; ST elevation & upright T wave in leads V_1 and V_2)
- rS or QS complex in right precordial leads

Note: Left axis deviation may be present (item 9c).

Note: LBBB interferes with determination of QRS axis and identification of ventricular hypertrophy and acute MI.

Note: Seen in:

- ▸ LVH
- ▸ MI
- ▸ Organic heart disease
- ▸ Congenital heart disease
- ▸ Degenerative conduction system disease
- ▸ Rarely in normals

7g. LBBB, intermittent

- Episodic LBBB (item 7f); more commonly seen at high rates (tachycardia-dependent) but may be bradycardia-dependent as well.

7h. Intraventricular conduction disturbance, nonspecific type

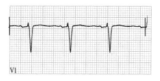

- QRS ≥ 0.11 seconds in duration but morphology does not meet criteria for LBBB (item 7f) or RBBB (item 7g), *or*

- Abnormal notching of the QRS complex without prolongation

Note: IVCD may be seen with:

  ‣ Antiarrhythmic drug toxicity (especially Type IA and IC agents) (item 14d)

  ‣ Hyperkalemia (item 14e)

  ‣ LVH (item 10a)

  ‣ Wolff-Parkinson-White (item 6h)

  ‣ Hypothermia (item 14u)

  ‣ Severe metabolic disturbances

7i. Aberrant intraventricular conduction with supraventricular arrhythmia

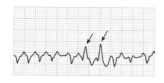

- Wide (> 0.12 seconds) QRS complex rhythm due to underlying supraventricular arrhythmia, such as atrial fibrillation, atrial flutter, other SVTs. May resemble VT (see item 4f for criteria to distinguish between SVT with aberrancy vs. VT).

Note: Return to normal intraventricular conduction may be accompanied by T wave abnormalities (item 12h).

P Wave Abnormalities

8a. Right atrial abnormality

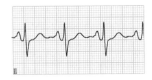

- Tall upright P wave:
  - ▸ > 2.5 mm in leads II, III, and aVF (P-pulmonale), *or*
  - ▸ > 1.5 mm in leads V_1 or V_2
- P wave axis shifted rightward (i.e., axis $\geq 70°$)

Note: In up to 30% of cases, P pulmonale may actually represent left atrial enlargement. Suspect this possibility when left atrial abnormality (item 8b) is present in lead V_1.

Note: Prominent atrial repolarization waves (Ta) can mimic Q waves and ST depression by deforming the PR and ST segments, respectively.

Note: P pulmonale can be seen in

- ▸ COPD with or without cor pulmonale
- ▸ Pulmonary hypertension

- ▸ Congenital heart disease (such as pulmonic stenosis, Tetralogy of Fallot, tricuspid atresia, Eisemenger's physiology)

- ▸ Pulmonary embolism (usually transient)

- ▸ Normal variant in patients with a thin body habitus and/or verticle heart

8b. Left atrial abnormality

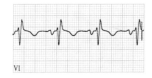

- Terminal negative portion of the P wave in lead $V_1 \geq 1$ mm deep and ≥ 0.04 seconds in duration (i.e., one small box deep and one small box wide), *or*

- Notched P wave with a duration ≥ 0.12 seconds in leads II, III or aVF (P-mitrale)

Note: Left atrial enlargement can exist with a normal P wave, and P mitrale may be present in the absence of left atrial enlargement.

Note: Prominent atrial repolarization waves (Ta) can mimic Q waves and ST depression by deforming the PR and ST segments, respectively.

Note: Mechanisms responsible for P mitrale include left atrial hypertrophy or dilation, intraatrial conduction delay, increased left atrial volume, and an acute rise in left atrial pressure.

8b-8c

<u>Note:</u> Can be seen in:

- ► Mitral valve disease
- ► Organic heart disease
- ► Aortic valve disease
- ► CHF
- ► MI

8c. Bi-atrial enlargement

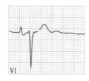

- Large biphasic P wave in $V_1 \geq 0.04$ seconds with:
  - ► An initial positive amplitude > 1.5 mm, *and*
  - ► A terminal negative amplitude ≥ 1 mm
- Tall peaked P waves (>1.5 mm) in the right precordial leads (V_1-V_3) and wide notched P waves in the left precordial leads (V_5-V_6)
- P wave amplitude ≥ 2.5 mm in the limb leads with a duration ≥ 0.12 seconds

8d. Nonspecific atrial abnormality

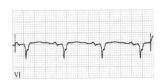

- Abnormal P wave morphology not fulfilling criteria for right (item 8a) or left atrial abnormality (item 8b)

QRS Voltage or Axis

9a. Low voltage, limb leads only

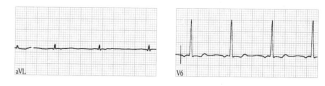

- Amplitude of the entire QRS complex (R+S) < 5 mm in all limb leads

Note: See item 9b for causes.

9b. Low voltage, limb and precordial leads

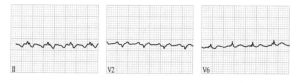

9b-9c

- Amplitude of the entire QRS complex (R+S) < 10 mm in each precordial lead, *and*
- Amplitude of R+S < 5 mm in all limb leads

Note: Causes include:

- ▸ Chronic lung disease (item 14m)
- ▸ Pericardial effusion (item 14o)
- ▸ Obesity
- ▸ Restrictive or infiltrative cardiomyopathies
- ▸ Coronary disease with extensive infarction of the left ventricle
- ▸ Myxedema (item 14t)
- ▸ Pleural effusion

9c. Left axis deviation

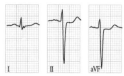

- Mean QRS axis between -30° and -90°

Note: Causes include:

- ▸ Left anterior fascicular block (if axis > -45°, item 7c)
- ▸ Inferior wall MI (item 11e, k)
- ▸ LBBB (item 7f)
- ▸ LVH (items 10 a, b)
- ▸ Ostium primum ASD (item 14j)

- ▸ COPD (item 14m)

- ▸ Hyperkalemia (item 14e)

9d. Right axis deviation

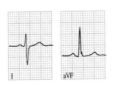

- • Mean QRS axis between 100° and 270°

- • Pure right axis deviation (left posterior fascicular block) should have an S wave in lead I and a Q wave in lead III (S_1 Q_3 pattern)

Note: Causes include:

- ▸ RVH (item 10c)

- ▸ Vertical heart

- ▸ Chronic obstructive pulmonary disease (item 14m)

- ▸ Pulmonary embolus (item 14n)

- ▸ Left posterior fascicular block (item 7d)

- ▸ Lateral wall myocardial infarction (items 11d, j)

- ▸ Dextrocardia (item 14k)

- ▸ Lead reversal (item 1c)

- ▸ Ostium secundum ASD (item 14i)

9e. Electrical alternans

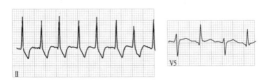

- Alternation in the amplitude and/or direction of P, QRS, and/or T waves

Note: Causes include:

  ▸ Pericardial effusion (item 14o)

     Note: Only one-third of patients with QRS alternans have a pericardial effusion. If electrical alternans involves the P-QRS-T ["total alternans"], effusion with tamponade is often present. Yet, only 12% of patients with pericardial effusions have electrical alternans.

  ▸ Severe left ventricular failure

  ▸ Hypertension

  ▸ Coronary artery disease

  ▸ Rheumatic heart disease

  ▸ Supraventricular or ventricular tachycardia

  ▸ Deep respirations

Note: Sizeable pericardial effusions electrically "insulate" the heart and result in low QRS voltage on the surface ECG. Electrical alternans, commonly associated with pericardial effusion, is due to swinging of the heart in the pericardial fluid during the cardiac cycle. If the pericardial effusion progresses to cardiac tamponade with overt or pending hemodynamic collapse, sinus tachycardia is almost always present.

Ventricular Hypertrophy

10a. Left ventricular hypertrophy by voltage only

- **Cornell Criteria** (most accurate):

  R wave in aVL + S wave in V_3:

  - ▸ > 24 mm in males
  - ▸ > 20 mm in females

- **Other commonly used voltage-based criteria**

  - ▸ **PRECORDIAL LEADS** (one or more)

    (1) R wave in V_5 or V_6 + S wave in V_1

    - ▸ > 35 mm if age > 30 years
    - ▸ > 40 mm if age 20-30 years
    - ▸ > 60 mm if age 16-19 years

    (2) Maximum R wave + S wave in precordial leads > 45 mm

    (3) R wave in V_5 > 26 mm

    (4) R wave in V_6 > 20 mm

  - ▸ **LIMB LEADS** (one or more)

    (1) R wave in lead I + S wave in lead II ≥ 26 mm

    (2) R wave in lead I ≥ 14 mm

    (3) S wave in aVR ≥ 15 mm

(4) R wave in aVL $\geq$ 12 mm (a highly specific finding, except when associated with left anterior fascicular block)

(5) R wave in aVF $\geq$ 21 mm

Note: The amplitude of the QRS (and sensitivity for the diagnosis of LVH by voltage criteria) is often decreased by conditions that increase the amount of body tissue (obesity), air (COPD, pneumothorax), fluid (pericardial or plural effusion), or fibrous tissue (coronary artery disease, sarcoid or amyloid of the heart) between the myocardium and ECG electrodes. Severe RVH can also underestimate the ECG diagnosis of LVH by canceling prominent QRS forces from the thickened LV. Left bundle branch block may also reduce QRS amplitude as well. In contrast, thin body habitus, left mastectomy, LBBB, WPW, and left anterior fascicular block may increase QRS amplitude in the absence of LVH, decreasing the specificity of the voltage criteria.

- **NON-VOLTAGE RELATED CRITERIA FOR LVH** (often seen with or without prominent voltage and ST-T changes in patients with LVH)

  - Left atrial abnormality (item 8b)
  - Left axis deviation (item 9c)
  - Nonspecific intraventricular conduction delay (item 7h)
  - Delayed onset of intrinsicoid deflection (beginning of QRS to peak of R wave > 0.05 seconds)
  - Small or absent R waves in V_1-V_3 (low anterior forces)
  - Absent Q waves in leads I, V_5, V_6
  - Abnormal Q waves in leads II, III, aVF (due to left axis deviation)

- ▸ Prominent U waves (item 12l)
- ▸ R wave in $V_6 > V_5$, provided there are dominant R waves in these leads

10b. LVH by voltage and ST-T segment abnormalities

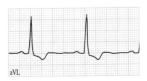

- • Voltage criteria for LVH (item 10a)
- • ST-T segment abnormalities (one or more):
  - ▸ ST segment and T wave deviation opposite in direction to the major deflection of QRS, usually manifesting as ST segment depression in leads I, aVL, III, aVF and/or V_4-V_6, and ST elevation ($< 0.5 - 3$ mm) in leads V_1-V_3
  - ▸ Inverted T waves in leads I, aVL, V_4-V_6
  - ▸ Prominent or inverted U waves

Note: Repolarization abnormalities associated with LVH are often mistaken for lateral myocardial ischemia (i.e., lateral ST depression and T wave inversions) and/or anterior/inferior myocardial infarction (i.e., Q waves in II, III, aVF, V_1-V_2, and ST elevation in V_1 - V_2). However, the presence of LVH with a "strain" pattern does not exclude superimposed ischemia.

Note: LVH (hypertensive heart disease) is probably the most common cause for false positive exercise treadmill ECG tests.

10c

10c. Right ventricular hypertrophy

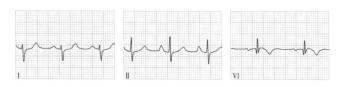

- Right axis deviation with mean QRS axis $\geq + 100°$
- Dominant R wave
  - R/S ratio in V_1 or $V_{3R} > 1$, *or* R/S ratio in V_5 or $V_6 \leq 1$
  - R wave in $V_1 \geq 7$mm
  - R wave in V_1 + S wave in V_5 or $V_6 > 10.5$ mm
  - rSR' in V_1 with R' > 10 mm
  - qR complex in V_1
- Secondary ST-T changes (downsloping ST depression, T-wave inversion) in right precordial leads
- Right atrial abnormality (item 8a)
- Onset of intrinsicoid deflection in V_1 between 0.035 and 0.055 seconds

Note: For ECG features of RVH in the setting of chronic lung disease, see item 14m.

Note: Severe RVH can also underestimate the ECG diagnosis of LVH by canceling prominent QRS forces from the thickened LV.

Note: Conditions that can present with right axis deviation and/or a dominant R wave and possibly mimic RVH include:

- Posterior or inferoposterolateral wall MI (item 11f). When a tall R wave is present in lead V_1, other ECG findings can help distinguish right ventricular hypertrophy (RVH) from posterior MI: T wave inversions in V_1V_2 and right axis deviation favors the diagnosis of RVH, while inferior Q waves suggestive of inferior MI favors the diagnosis of posterior MI.

▸ Right bundle branch block (item 7b)

▸ Wolff-Parkinson-White syndrome (type A) (item 6h)

▸ Dextrocardia (item 14k)

▸ Left posterior fascicular block (item 7d)

▸ Normal variant (especially in children)

10d. Combined ventricular hypertrophy

Suggested by any of the following:

- ECG meets one or more diagnostic criteria for both isolated LVH (item 10a, b) and RVH (item 10c)

- Precordial leads show LVH but QRS axis is >90°

- LVH *plus:*

    ▸ R wave > Q wave in aVR, *and*

    ▸ S wave > R wave in V_5, *and*

    ▸ T wave inversion in V_1

- Large amplitude, equiphasic (R=S) complexes in V_3 and V_4 (Kutz-Wachtel phenomenon)

- Right atrial abnormality (item 8a) with LVH pattern (item 10a, b) in precordial leads

Q Wave Myocardial Infarction

- **MYOCARDIAL ISCHEMIA VS. INJURY VS. INFARCTION**

    ‣ Ischemia: ST segment depression: T waves usually inverted; Q waves absent

    ‣ Injury: ST segment elevation; Q waves absent

    ‣ Infarction: Abnormal Q waves; ST segment elevation or depression; T waves inverted, normal, or upright & symmetrically peaked

    <u>Note</u>: Exception: MI may be present without Q waves in:

    - Anterior MI: May only see low anterior R wave forces with decreasing R wave progression in leads V_2-V_5

    - Posterior MI: Dominant R wave and ST depression in leads V_1-V_3

- **SIGNIFICANT ST ELEVATION**

    ‣ $\geq$ 1-2 mm in two or more contiguous leads

    ‣ Usually with upwardly convex configuration

    ‣ Can persist 48 hours to 4 weeks after MI

    <u>Note:</u> Persistent ST elevation beyond 4 weeks suggests the presence of a ventricular aneurysm (item 11m)

- **T WAVE INVERSION** typically begins while the ST segments are still elevated (in contrast to pericarditis) and may persist indefinitely

    <u>Note:</u> Acute infarction can occur without significant ST segment elevation or depression: up to 40% of patients with acute occlusion of the left circumflex coronary artery and 10-

15% of patients with RCA or LAD occlusions may not have significant ECG changes.

- **ABNORMAL Q WAVES**

  ‣ Duration $\geq$ 0.03-0.04 seconds for most leads

  ‣ Duration $\geq$ 0.04 seconds in leads III, aVL, aVF, and V_1

  Note: The presence of a Q wave cannot be used to reliably distinguish transmural from subendocardial MI.

  Note: Abnormal Q waves regress or disappear over months to years in up to 20% of patients with Q-wave MI.

- **AGE OF INFARCT CAN BE APPROXIMATED FROM THE ECG:**

  ‣ <u>Probably Acute or Recent MI:</u> The repolarization abnormalities associated with acute myocardial infarction typically evolve in a relatively predictable fashion. Usually, the earliest finding is marked peaking of the T waves ("<u>hyperacute T waves</u>") in the region of the infarct; these are often missed since they occur very early (< 15 minutes) in the course of the acute event and are transient. If transmural ischemia persists for more than a few minutes, the peaked T waves evolve into <u>ST segment elevation</u>, which should be $\geq$ 1 mm in height to be considered significant. The ST segment elevation of myocardial infarction is usually upwardly *convex* (in contrast to acute pericarditis or normal variant early repolarization, in which the ST elevation is usually upwardly *concave)*. As the acute infarction continues to evolve, the ST segment elevation decreases and the <u>T waves begin to invert</u>. The T waves usually become progressively deeper as the ST segment elevation subsides. <u>Abnormal Q waves</u> develop within the first few hours to days after an infarction.

11

- Acute MI: Abnormal Q waves, ST elevation (associated ST depression is sometimes present in noninfarct leads)

- Recent MI: Abnormal Q waves, isoelectric ST segments, ischemic (usually inverted) T waves

▸ <u>Probably old or age indeterminate MI:</u> Abnormal Q waves, isoelectric ST segments, nonspecific or normal T waves

<u>Note</u>: Exception: MI may be present without Q waves in:

- Anterior MI: May only see low anterior R wave forces with decreasing R wave progression in leads V_2-V_5

- Posterior MI: Dominant R wave and ST depression in leads V_1-V_3

- **PSEUDOINFARCTION PATTERN:** Conditions causing "pseudoinfarcts" (ECG pattern mimicking myocardial infarction) include:

▸ Wolff-Parkinson-White (item 6h): Negative delta waves mimic Q waves

▸ Hypertrophic cardiomyopathy (item 14q): Q waves in I, aVL, V_4-V_6 due to septal hypertrophy

▸ LVH (items 10a, b): Poor R wave progression, at times with ST elevation in V_1-V_3, can mimic anteroseptal MI. Inferior Q waves may be present and can mimic inferior MI

▸ LBBB (item 7f): QS pattern in V_1-V_4 mimics anteroseptal MI. Less commonly, Q waves in III and aVF mimic inferior MI

▸ RVH (item 10c)

— 124 —

- Left anterior fascicular block (item 7c)
- Chronic lung disease (item 14m): Q waves appear in inferior and/or right and mid-precordial leads
- Amyloid, sarcoid, and other Infiltrative diseases: Electrically active tissue replaced by inert substance
- Cardiomyopathy
- Chest deformity (e.g., pectus excavatum)
- Pulmonary embolism (item 14n): Q wave in lead III and sometimes aVF, but Q waves in II are rare
- Myocarditis
- Myocardial tumors
- Hyperkalemia (item 14g)
- Pneumothorax: QS complex in right precordial leads
- Pancreatitis
- Lead reversal (item 1c)
- Corrected transposition
- Muscular dystrophy
- Mitral valve prolapse: Rare Q wave in III and aVF
- Myocardial contusion: Q waves in areas of intramyocardial hemorrhage and edema
- Left/right atrial enlargement: Prominent atrial repolarization wave (Ta) can depress the PR segment and mimic Q waves
- Atrial flutter (item 2x): Flutter waves may deform the PR segment and simulate Q waves
- Dextrocardia (item 14k)

11a-11c

- **DIAGNOSIS OF Q WAVE MI IN THE PRESENCE OF BUNDLE BRANCH BLOCK**
  - ▸ RBBB: Does not interfere with the diagnosis of Q wave MI; Q wave criteria apply for all infarctions
  - ▸ LBBB: Difficult to diagnose any infarct in the presence of LBBB. However, acute injury is sometimes apparent (item 7e)

11a. Anterolateral MI, recent or probably acute

- Abnormal Q waves (duration $\geq$ 0.03 seconds) in leads V_4-V_6, *accompanied by*
- ST segment elevation

11b. Anterior MI, recent or probably acute

- rS in V_1, *followed by*
  - ▸ QS or QR complexes (Q wave duration $\geq$ 0.03 seconds) V_4, *or* accompanied by decreasing R wave amplitude from V_2-V_5
- ST segment elevation (in the of leads V_2-V_4).

11c. Anteroseptal MI, recent or probably acute

- Abnormal Q or QS deflection in V_1-V_3 and sometimes V_4 (Q wave duration $\geq$ 0.04 seconds in V_1 and $\geq$ 0.03 seconds in V_2-V_4), *accompanied by*
- ST segment elevation

Note: The presence of a Q wave in V_1 distinguishes anteroseptal from anterior infarction.

11d. Lateral/high lateral MI, recent or probably acute

- Abnormal Q wave in lead I (duration ≥ 0.03 seconds) and aVL (duration ≥ 0.04 seconds), *accompanied by*
- ST segment elevation

<u>Note:</u> An isolated Q wave in aVL does not qualify as a lateral MI.

11e. Inferior MI, recent or probably acute

- Abnormal Q waves in at least two of leads II, III, aVF (Q wave duration ≥ 0.03 seconds in lead II and ≥ 0.04 seconds in leads III and aVF), *accompanied by*
- ST segment elevation

<u>Note:</u> Associated ST depression is usually evident in leads I, aVL, V_1-V_3.

11f. Posterior MI, recent or probably acute

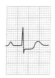

- Initial R wave ≥ 0.04 seconds in V_1 and V_2 with:
  - R wave ≥ S wave, *and*
  - ST segment depression (usually ≥ 2 mm) with upright T waves

11f-11k

<u>Note:</u> The posterior wall of the left ventricular differs from the anterior, inferior, and lateral walls by not having ECG leads directly overly it. Instead of Q waves and ST elevation, acute posterior MI presents with mirror-image changes in the anterior precordial leads (V_1-V_3), including dominant R waves (the mirror-image of abnormal Q waves), and horizontal ST segment depression (the mirror-image of ST elevation). Acute posterior infarction is often associated with ECG changes of acute inferior or inferolateral myocardial infarction, but may occur in isolation. <u>Note:</u> RVH (item 10c), WPW (item 6h), and RBBB (item 7b) may interfere with the ECG diagnosis of posterior MI.

11g. Anterolateral MI, age indeterminate or old

- See item 11a, no ST segment elevation

11h. Anterior MI, age indeterminate or old

- See item 11b, no ST segment elevation

11i. Anteroseptal MI, age indeterminate or old

- See item 11c, no ST segment elevation

11j. Lateral/high lateral MI, age indeterminate or old

- See item 11d, no ST segment elevation

11k. Inferior infarct, age indeterminate or old

- See item 11e, no ST segment elevation

11l. Posterior MI, age indeterminate or old

- See item 11f, no ST segment depression characteristic of acute posterior injury

11m. Probable ventricular aneurysm

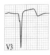

- ST segment elevation ≥ 1 mm persisting 4 or more weeks after acute MI in leads with abnormal Q waves

Note: The ST elevation of ventricular aneurysm differs from pericarditis in several ways: In ventricular aneurysm, ST elevation is localized, Q waves are usually present in the same leads with ST elevation, and ST and T wave changes remain stable over time. In pericarditis, ST elevation is diffuse, Q waves are not evident (unless pericarditis follows acute MI), and ST and T wave changes evolve and are transient.

Note: Anteroseptal infarction accounts for approximately of 80% of the aneurysms noted after myocardial infarction, and posterior infarction accounts for the other 20%.

12a-12b

ST, T, U Wave

12a. Normal variant, early repolarization

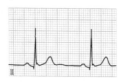

- Elevated take-off of ST segment at the junction between the QRS and ST segment (J junction)
- Concave upward ST elevation ending with a symmetrical upright T wave (often of large amplitude)
- Distinct notch or slur on downstroke of R wave
- Most commonly involves V_2-V_5; sometimes II, III, aVF
- No reciprocal ST segment depression

Note: Some degree of ST elevation is present in the majority of young healthy individuals, especially in the precordial leads.

12b. Normal variant, juvenile T waves

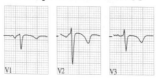

- Persistently negative T waves (usually not symmetrical or deep) in leads V_1-V_3 in normal adults

- T waves still upright I, II, V_5, V_6

Note: Juvenile T waves is a normal variant ECG finding commonly seen in children, occasionally seen as a normal variant in adult women, but only rarely seen in adult men.

12c. Nonspecific ST and/or T wave abnormalities

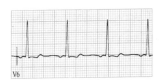

- Slight (< 1mm) ST depression or elevation, *and/or*
- T wave flat or slightly inverted

Note: Normal T waves usually ≥ 10% the height of R wave

Note: Can be seen in:

- ‣ Organic heart disease
- ‣ Drugs (e.g., quinidine)
- ‣ Electrolyte disorders (e.g., hypokalemia, item 14f)
- ‣ Hyperventilation
- ‣ Hypothyroidism (item 14t)
- ‣ Stress
- ‣ Pancreatitis
- ‣ Pericarditis (item 14p)
- ‣ CNS disorders (item 14s)

12c-12d

- ‣ LVH (item 10b)
- ‣ RVH (item 10c)
- ‣ Bundle branch block (items 7a, f)
- ‣ Healthy adults (normal variant) (item 1b)
- ‣ Persistent juvenile pattern: T wave inversion in V_1-V_3 in young adults

12d. ST and/or T wave abnormalities suggesting myocardial ischemia

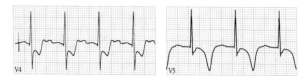

- • Ischemic ST segment changes:
  - ‣ Horizontal or downsloping ST segments with or without T wave inversion

  <u>Note:</u> Flutter waves or prominent atrial repolarization waves (as can be seen in left/right atrial enlargement, pericarditis, atrial infarction) can deform the ST segment and result in "pseudodepression."

- • Ischemic T wave changes:
  - ‣ Biphasic T waves with or without ST depression
  - ‣ Symmetrical or deeply inverted T waves; QT interval is usually prolonged.
  - ‣ Hyperacute T waves

Note: Reciprocal T wave changes may be evident (e.g., tall upright T waves in inferior leads with deeply inverted T waves in anterior leads).

Note: T waves may become less inverted or upright during acute ischemia ("pseudonormalization").

Note: Prominent U waves (upright or inverted) (item 12l) are often present.

Note: Tall upright T waves may also be seen in:

- ▸ Normal healthy adults (item 1b)
- ▸ Hyperkalemia (item 14e)
- ▸ Early MI
- ▸ LVH (item 10b)
- ▸ CNS disorders (item 14s)
- ▸ Anemia

12e. ST-T wave changes suggesting myocardial injury

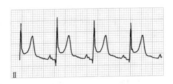

- Acute ST segment elevation with upward convexity in the leads representing the area of infarction

- ST & T wave changes evolve: T waves invert before ST segments return to baseline

- Associated ST depression in the noninfarct leads is common

12e-12f

- Acute posterior wall injury often has horizontal or downsloping ST segment depression with upright T waves in V_1-V_3, with or without a prominent R wave in these same leads

Note: ST & T wave changes suggesting myocardial injury can also be seen in:

- ▸ Post-tachycardia sinus beats (T wave inversion) (item 12h)
- ▸ Apical hypertrophic cardiomyopathy (item 14q)
- ▸ Central nervous system disease (item 14s)

12f. ST-T wave changes suggesting acute pericarditis

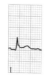 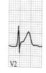 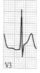

- Classic evolutionary pattern consists of 4 stages (but is not always present):
  - ▸ Stage 1: Upwardly concave ST segment elevation in almost all leads except aVR; no reciprocal ST depression in other leads except aVR
  - ▸ Stage 2: ST junction (J point) returns to baseline and T wave amplitude begins to decrease
  - ▸ Stage 3: T waves invert
  - ▸ Stage 4: ECG returns to normal

Note: T wave inversion occurs *after* the ST segment returns to baseline (in contrast to myocardial infarction, where T wave inversion typically begins while the ST segments are still elevated).

- Other clues to acute pericarditis (item 14p):

    ▸ Sinus tachycardia (item 2d)

    ▸ PR depression early (PR elevation in aVR)

    ▸ Low voltage QRS (item 8b)

    ▸ Electrical alternans (item 9e) if pericardial effusion (item 14o)

Note: Pericarditis may be focal (e.g., post-pericardiotomy) and result in regional (rather than diffuse) ST elevation.

Note: Classic ST and T wave changes are more likely to occur in purulent pericarditis as opposed to idiopathic, rheumatic, or malignant pericarditis.

12g. ST and/or T wave changes secondary to IVCD or hypertrophy

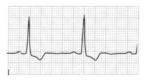

- *LVH:* ST segment and T wave displacement opposite to the major QRS deflection:

    ▸ ST depression (upwardly concave) & T wave inversion when the QRS is mainly positive (leads I, V_5, V_6)

> ‣ Subtle (< 1 mm) ST elevation and upright T waves when the QRS is mainly negative (leads V_1, V_2)

- **RVH:** ST segment depression and T wave inversion in leads V_1-V_3 and sometimes in leads II, III, aVF

- **LBBB:** ST segment and T wave displacement opposite to the major QRS deflection

- **RBBB:** Uncomplicated RBBB has little ST displacement. T wave vector is opposite to the terminal slurred portion of QRS (upright in leads I, V_5, V_6; inverted in leads V_1, V_2)

12h. Post-extrasystolic T wave abnormality

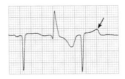

- Any alternation in contour, amplitude and/or direction of the T wave in the sinus beat(s) following ectopic or ventricular paced beat(s)

12i. Isolated J point depression

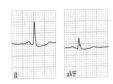

- ST segment depression ≥ 1 mm at the junction of the QRS and ST segment (J-point) lasting ≥ 0.08 seconds

Note: Most frequently seen during exercise testing.

12j. Peaked T waves

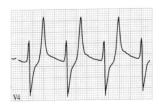

- T wave > 6 mm in limb leads, *or*
- T wave > 10 mm in precordial leads

Note: Causes of peaked T waves include:

- ▸ Acute MI (item 12e)
- ▸ Angina pectoris

12j-12k

- ▸ Normal variant (item 1b): usually effects mid-precordial leads

- ▸ Hyperkalemia (item 14e): more common when the rise in serum potassium is acute

- ▸ Intracranial bleeding (item 14s)

- ▸ LVH (item 10b)

- ▸ RVH (item 10c)

- ▸ LBBB (item 7f)

- ▸ Superimposed P wave: from APC, sinus rhythm with marked first-degree AV block, complete heart block, etc.

- ▸ Anemia

12k. Prolonged QT interval

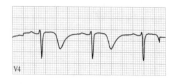

- • Corrected QT inteval (QTc) ≥ 0.44 seconds, where $QTc = QT$ *interval divided by the square root of the preceding RR interval*

Note: Be sure to measure the QT interval in a lead with a large T wave and distinct termination. Also look for the lead with the longest QT.

- Easier methods to determine QT interval:

  ▸ Use 0.40 seconds as the normal QT interval for a heart rate of 70. For every 10 BPM change in heart rate above (or below) 70, subtract (or add) 0.02 seconds. (Measured value should be within ±0.07 seconds of the calculated normal.) <u>Example:</u> For a HR of 100 BPM, the calculated "normal" QT interval = 0.34 ± .07 seconds (0.40 sec - 3 [0.02 sec]). For a HR of 50 BPM, the calculated "normal" QT interval = 0.44 ± .07 seconds (0.40 sec + 2 [0.02 sec]).

  ▸ The normal QT interval should be less than 50% of the RR interval

Note: The QT interval represents the period of ventricular electrical systole (i.e., the time required for ventricular depolarization and repolarization to occur), varies inversely with heart rate, and is longer while asleep than while awake (presumably due to vagal hypertonia).

Note: Conditions associated with a prolonged QT interval include:
- ▸ Drugs (quinidine, procainamide, disopyramide, amiodarone, sotalol, phenothiazine, tricyclics, lithium) (item 14c, d)

- ▸ Hypomagnesemia

- ▸ Hypocalcemia (item 14h)

- ▸ Marked bradyarrhythmias
- ▸ Intracranial hemorrhage (item 14s)
- ▸ Myocarditis
- ▸ Mitral valve prolapse
- ▸ Hypothyroidism (item 14t)
- ▸ Hypothermia (item 14u)
- ▸ Liquid protein diets
- ▸ Romano-Ward syndrome (congenital; normal hearing)
- ▸ Jervell and Lange-Nielson syndrome (congential; deafness)

12l. Prominent U waves

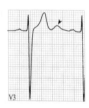

- • Amplitude ≥ 1.5 mm

  <u>Note:</u> The U wave is normally 5-25% the height of the T wave, and is largest in leads V_2 and V_3

  <u>Note:</u> Causes include:

- ▸ Hypokalemia (item 14f)
- ▸ Bradyarrhythmias
- ▸ Hypothermia (item 14u)
- ▸ LVH (item 10b)
- ▸ Coronary artery disease
- ▸ Drugs (digitalis, quinidine, amiodarone, isoproterenol) (items 14a, c)

12m. Poor R Wave Progression

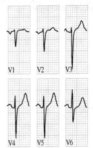

- Lead with equal positive and negative deflection (or lead where R wave amplitude exceeds S wave amplitude) = V_5 or V_6
- Can be seen in:
  - Normals
  - Anteroseptal or anterior MI (items 11c, b)

- Dilated or hypertrophic cardiomyopathy
- LVH (item 10b)
- COPD (item 14m)
- Cor pulmonale (item 14n)
- RVH (item 10c)
- Left anterior fascicular block (item 7c)

Pacemakers

13a. Atrial or coronary sinus pacing

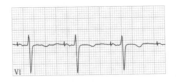

- Pacemaker stimulus followed by an atrial depolarization
- If the rate of the intrinsic rhythm falls below that of the pacemaker, atrial paced beats occur and will be separated by a constant (A-A) interval.
- Appropriately sensed intrinsic atrial activity (P wave) resets pacemaker timing clock. After an interval of time (A-A

interval) with no sensed atrial activity, an atrial paced beat occurs.

13b. Ventricular demand pacing

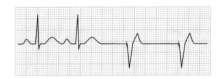

- Pacemaker stimulus followed by a QRS complex of different morphology than intrinsic QRS

- A ventricular demand (VVI) pacemaker senses and paces only in the ventricle and is oblivious to native atrial activity. If constant ventricular pacing is noted throughout the tracing, it is impossible to distinguish ventricular demand from asynchronous ventricular pacing. Thus, the diagnosis of ventricular demand pacing requires evidence of appropriate inhibition of pacemaker output in response to a native QRS (at least one).

- Appropriately sensed ventricular activity (QRS complex) resets pacemaker timing clock. After an interval of time (V-V interval) with no sensed ventricular activity, a ventricular paced beat is delivered and a new cycle begins.

- A spontaneous QRS arising before the end of the V-V interval is sensed and the ventricular output of the pacemaker is inhibited. A new timing cycle begins.

- For rate-responsive VVI-R pacemakers, ventricular paced rate increases with activity (up to a defined upper rate limit).

13c. Ventricular pacing, fixed rate (asynchronous)

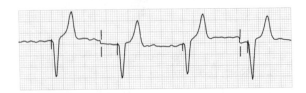

- Ventricular pacing with no demonstrable output inhibition by intrinsic QRS complexes

<u>Note:</u> Ventricular pacing should be considered the equivalent of LBBB when it comes to identifying acute myocardial infarction. Ventricular pacing results in an abnormal ventricular activation pattern, resulting in wide QRS complexes with secondary ST-T abnormalities; this makes the diagnosis of acute myocardial ischemia and/or infarction extremely difficult unless portions of the ECG show unpaced QRS complexes.

<u>Note:</u> This relatively uncommon pacing mode (i.e., VOO) can be mistaken as pacemaker malfunction — failure to sense.

13d. AV sequential pacing

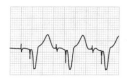

- Atrial followed by ventricular pacing

- Could be DVI, DDD, DDI, or DOO pacing mode

13e. Dual chamber, atrial-sensing pacemaker

- For atrial sensing, need to demonstrate inhibition of atrial output and/or triggering of ventricular stimulus in response to intrinsic atrial depolarization

- If pacemaker rate exceeds rate of intrinsic rhythm, there will be atrial (A) and ventricular (V) paced beats with defined intervals between the A and V spikes (A-V interval) and from the V spike to the subsequent A spike (V-A interval);

- Following V sensed activity (either QRS or paced [V] beats), the timing clock is reset. If intrinsic atrial activity (P) is sensed prior to the end of the V-A interval, an atrial output of the pacemaker will be inhibited. If no intrinsic atrial activity (P) is sensed by the end of the V-A interval, an atrial paced beat will occur.

13e-13f

- Following atrial sensed activity (either intrinsic (P) or paced (A) beats), the timing clock is reset. If intrinsic ventricular activity (QRS) is sensed prior to the end of the AV interval, ventricular output of the pacemaker will be inhibited. If no intrinsic ventricular activity (QRS) is sensed by the end of the A-V interval, a ventricular paced beat will occur.

13f. Pacemaker malfunction, not constantly capturing (atrium or ventricle)

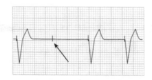

- Pacing spike is not followed by appropriate depolarization (at a time when myocardium is not refractory).

- May be due to lead displacement, perforation, increased pacing threshold (from MI, flecainide, amiodarone, hyperkalemia), lead fracture or insulation break, pulse generator failure (from battery depletion), or inappropriate reprogramming.

Note: Rule out "pseudo-malfunction" (i.e., pacer stimulus falls into refractory period of ventricle)

13g. Pacemaker malfunction, not constantly sensing

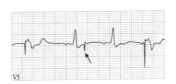

- Pacemakers in Inhibited Mode: Failure of pacemaker to be inhibited by an appropriate intrinsic depolarization

- Pacemakers in Triggered Mode: Failure of pacemaker to be triggered by an appropriate intrinsic depolarization

- Pacemaker timing is not rest by intrinsic or ectopic beat, resulting in asynchronous firing of pacemaker (paced rhythm competes with the intrinsic rhythm)

- Occurs with low amplitude signals (esp. VPCs) and inappropriate programming of the sensitivity. All causes of failure to capture (item 13f) can also cause fail to sense.

<u>Note:</u> Can often be corrected by reprogramming the sensitivity of the pacemaker.

<u>Note:</u> Watch for "pseudo-malfunction" (i.e., pacer stimulus falls into refractory period of ventricle)

<u>Note:</u> Premature depolarizations may not be sensed if they:

  ‣ Fall within the programmed refractory period of the pacemaker

13g-13j

> ▸ Have insufficient amplitude at the sensing electrode site

Note: Any stimulus falling within the QRS complex probably does not represent sensing malfunction (commonly seen with right ventricular electrodes in RBBB).

13h. Pacemaker malfunction, not firing

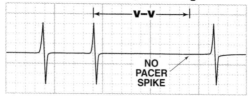

• Failure of appropriate pacemaker output

13i. Pacemaker malfunction, slowing

• Increase in stimulus intervals over the programmed intervals

Note: Usually an indicator of battery end of life

Note: Often noted first during magnet application

13j. Oversensing of T waves

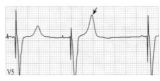

- Failure of pacemaker discharge at the appropriate time; caused by resetting of pacemaker clock by T waves (as well as P waves or myopotentials), which are mistaken for R waves. Ventricular stimulus escape (VA) interval is thus timed from the T wave.

  Note: Can be corrected by reprogramming the sensitivity or refractory period of the chamber that is oversensing.

13k. Oversensing due to myopotential inhibition

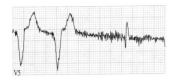

- Pacemaker inhibition by myopotentials (muscular potentials from arm movements) inappropriately sensed as cardiac potentials
- Paced RR intervals tend to be irregular

  Note: More common with unipolar pacemakers.

13l-13m

13l. Upper rate pacing

- Rapid pacing at or near upper rate limit of pacemaker

- Occurs in supraventricular tachycardia (e.g., atrial fibrillation) when frequent atrial depolarizations are sensed and tracked by a dual-chamber pacemaker.

  Note: Can be corrected by programming to VVI mode and/or conversion of the rhythm.

13m. Pacemaker-mediated tachycardia

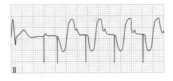

- Rapid pacing at or near upper rate limit of pacemaker occurs when retrograde atrial activity from ventricular paced beats is repetitively sensed in the atrium, triggering ventricular paced complexes in patients with dual chamber pacemakers with atrial sensing

  Note: Can usually be corrected by increasing the post-ventricular atrial refractory period (PVARP) of the pacemaker.

Clinical Disorders

14a. Digitalis effect

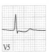

- Sagging ST segment depression with upward concavity

- T wave flat, inverted, or biphasic

- QT interval shortened

- U wave amplitude increased

- PR interval lengthened

Note: ST changes are difficult to interpret in the setting of LVH, RVH, or bundle branch block. However, if typical sagging ST segments are present and the QT interval is shortened, consider digitalis effect.

14b. Digitalis toxicity

- Digitalis toxicity can cause almost any type of cardiac dysrhythmia or conduction disturbance except bundle branch block. Typical abnormalities include:

  ‣ Paroxysmal atrial tachycardia with block (item 2o)

14b-14c

- Atrial fibrillation with complete heart block (regular RR intervals)

- Second or third-degree AV block (items 6b, c, e)

- Complete heart block (item 6e) with accelerated junctional rhythm (item 3c) or accelerated idioventricular rhythm (items 4g)

- Supraventricular tachycardia with alternating bundle branch block

Note: Digitalis toxicity may be exacerbated by hypokalemia, hypomagnesemia, and hypercalcemia.

Note: Electrical cardioversion of atrial fibrillation is contraindicated in the setting of digitalis toxicity since protracted asystole or ventricular fibrillation can occur. (Digitalis levels should always be checked prior to elective electrical cardioversion).

14c. Antiarrhythmic drug effect

Suggested by the following:

- Prolonged QT interval (item 12k)

- Prominent U waves (one of the earliest findings) (item 12l)

- Nonspecific ST and/or T wave changes (item 12c)

- Decrease in atrial flutter rate

14d. Antiarrhythmic drug toxicity

Suggested by the following:

- Prolonged QT (item 12k)

- Ventricular arrhythmias including "Torsade de Pointes" (paroxysms of irregular ventricular tachyarrhythmia at a rate of 200-280 BPM with sinusoidal cycles of changing QRS amplitude and polarity in the setting of a prolonged QT interval)

- Wide QRS complex

- Various degrees of AV block

- Marked sinus bradycardia (item 2c), sinus arrest (item 2e), or SA block (item 2f)

14e. Hyperkalemia

- $K^+ = 5.5 - 6.5$ mEq/L

  ‣ Tall, peaked, narrow based T waves

  ‣ QT interval shortening

  ‣ Reversible left anterior fascicular block (item 7c) or left posterior fascicular block (item 7d)

- $K^+ = 6.5 - 7.5$ mEq/L

  ‣ First-degree AV block (item 6a)

  ‣ Flattening and widening of the P wave

  ‣ ST segment depression

- ‣ QRS widening
- $K^+ > 7.5$ mEq/L
  - ‣ Disappearance of P waves, which may be caused by:
    - • Sinus arrest (item 2e), *or*
    - • "Sinoventricular conduction" (sinus impulses conducted to the ventricles via specialized atrial fibers *without* atrial depolarization)
  - ‣ LBBB (item 7f), RBBB (item 7b), or markedly widened and diffuse intraventricular conduction delay (item 7h) resembling a sine wave pattern
  - ‣ Arrhythmias and conduction disturbances including VT (item 4f), VF (item 4i), idioventricular rhythm, asystole

14f. Hypokalemia

Suggested by the following:

- Prominent U waves (item 12l)
- ST segment depression and flattened T waves

  Note: The ST-T and U wave changes of hypokalemia are seen in approximately 80% of patients with potassium levels < 2.7 mEq/L, compared to 35% of patients with levels of 2.7-3.0 mEq/L, and 10% of patients with levels >3.0 mEq/L.

- Increased amplitude and duration of the P wave
- Prolonged QT sometimes seen

Note: If potassium replacement does not normalize the QT interval, suspect hypomagnesemia.

- Arrhythmias and conduction disturbances including paroxysmal atrial tachycardia with block (item 2o), first-degree AV block (item 6a), Type I second-degree AV block (item 6b), AV dissociation (item 5d), VPCs (item 4a), ventricular tachycardia (item 4f), and ventricular fibrillation (item 4i).

14g. Hypercalcemia

- QTc shortening (usually due to shortening of the ST segment)
- May see PR prolongation

Note: Little if any effect on P, QRS, or T wave.

14h. Hypocalcemia

- Prolonged QTc (item 12k) (earliest and most common finding). Due to ST segment prolongation, which occurs without changing the duration of the T wave; only hypothermia and hypocalcemia do this.
- Occasional flattening, peaking, or inversion of T waves

14i-14j

14i. Atrial septal defect, ostium secundum

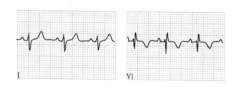

Suggested by the following:

- Typical RSR' or rSR' complex in V_1 with a QRS duration < 0.11 seconds

- Incomplete RBBB

- Right axis deviation (item 9d) ± right ventricular hypertrophy (item 10c)

- Right atrial abnormality (item 8a) in ~ 30%

- First-degree AV block (item 6a) in < 20%

<u>Note:</u> Ostium secundum ASDs represent 70% of all ASDs, and are due to deficient tissue in the region of the fossa ovalis.

14j. Atrial septal defect, ostium primum

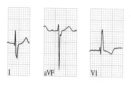

Suggested by the following:

- RSR' complex in V_1

- Incomplete RBBB

- Left axis deviation (in contrast to right axis deviation in ostium secundum ASD)

- First-degree AV block (item 6a) in 15-40%

- Advanced cases have biventricular hypertrophy (item 10d)

<u>Note:</u> Ostium primum ASDs represent 15% of all ASDs, and are due to deficient tissue in the lower portion of the septum. These ASDs are usually large, may be accompanied by anomalous pulmonary venous drainage, and are associated with a cleft anterior mitral valve leaflet, mitral regurgitation, and Down's syndrome.

14k. Dextrocardia, mirror image

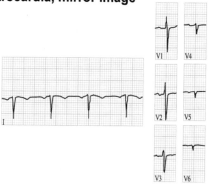

Suggested by the following:

- P-QRS-T in leads I and aVL are inverted or "upside down"

  Note: Dextrocardia and lead reversal (item 1c) can both produce an upside down P-QRS-T in leads I and aVL. To distinguish between these conditions, look at the R wave pattern in V_1 - V_6:

  ‣ Reverse R wave progression (i.e., decreasing R wave amplitude form leads V_1-V_6) suggests dextrocardia

  ‣ Normal R wave progression suggests lead reversal

Note: In *mirror-image dextrocardia*, the most common form of dextrocardia, the abdominal and thoracic viscera (in addition to the heart) are transposed to the side opposite their usual locations (dextrocardia with "situs inversus"). This form of dextrocardia is generally not associated with severe congenital cardiac abnormalities (other than the malposition, which does not affect cardiac function). In *isolated dextrocardia*, the heart is rotated to the right side of the chest but other viscera remain in their usual locations. This type of dextrocardia is almost always associated with serious congenital cardiac abnormalities, resulting in clinical difficulties in infancy or early childhood.

14l. Mitral valve disease

- Mitral stenosis

  ‣ Combination of right ventricular hypertrophy (item 10c) and left atrial abnormality (item 8b) is suggestive

- Mitral valve prolapse

    ‣ Flattened or inverted T waves in leads II, III and aVF (and sometimes in right precordial leads) ± ST segment depression, which is sometimes present in the left precordial leads

    ‣ Prominent U waves (item 12l)

    ‣ Prolonged QT interval (item 12k)

14m. Chronic lung disease

- ECG features suggestive of COPD include:

    ‣ Right ventricular hypertrophy (item 10c)

    ‣ Right axis deviation (item 9d)

    ‣ Right atrial abnormality (item 8a)

    ‣ Shift of transitional zone counterclockwise (poor R wave progression)

    ‣ Low voltage QRS (items 9a, b)

    ‣ Pseudo-anteroseptal infarct pattern (low anterior forces)

    ‣ S waves in leads I, II, and III ($S_1 S_2 S_3$ pattern)

- May also see sinus tachycardia (item 2d), junctional rhythm (item 3d), multifocal atrial tachycardia (item 2n), various degrees of AV block, IVCD (item 7h), and bundle branch block

14m-14n

<u>Note:</u> Right ventricular hypertrophy in the setting of chronic lung disease is suggested by:

- ▸ Rightward shift of QRS
- ▸ T wave inversion in V_1, V_2
- ▸ ST depression in leads II, III, aVF
- ▸ Transient RBBB
- ▸ RSR' or QR complex in V_1

14n. Acute cor pulmonale including pulmonary embolus

- ECG changes often accompany large pulmonary emboli and are associated with elevated pulmonary artery pressures, right ventricular dilation and strain, and clockwise rotation of the heart:

  - ▸ **$S_1 Q_3$ or $S_1 Q_3 T_3$** occurs in up to 30% of cases and lasts for 1-2 weeks

  - ▸ **Right bundle branch block** (incomplete or complete) may be seen in up to 25% of cases and usually lasts less than 1 week

  - ▸ **Inverted T waves** secondary to right ventricular strain may be seen in the right precordial leads and can last for months.

  - ▸ Other ECG findings include right axis deviation, nonspecific ST and T wave changes, and P pulmonale.

- ► Arrhythmias and conduction disturbances include sinus tachycardia (most common), atrial fibrillation, atrial flutter, atrial tachycardia, and first-degree AV block.

- The clinical presentation and ECG of acute pulmonary embolism may sometimes be confused with acute inferior MI: Q waves and T wave inversions may be seen in leads III and aVF in both conditions, however, a Q wave in lead II is uncommon in pulmonary embolism and suggests MI.

Note: ECG abnormalities are often *transient*, and a normal ECG may be recorded despite persistence of the embolus. Sinus tachycardia, however, is usually present even when other ECG features of acute cor pulmonale are absent.

14o. Pericardial effusion

- Low voltage QRS (item 9a, b) and/or electrical alternans (item 9e)

    Note: Low voltage QRS complexes and electrical alternans are consistent with (but not very sensitive or specific for) the diagnosis of pericardial effusion.

- Other features of acute pericarditis (item 12f) may or may not be present

14p. Acute pericarditis

- Refer to item 12f for criteria and ECG

14q

14q. Hypertrophic cardiomyopathy

- Majority have abnormal QRS

  - Large amplitude QRS

  - Large abnormal Q waves (can give pseudoinfarct pattern in inferior, lateral, and anterior precordial leads)

  - Tall R wave with inverted T wave in V_1 simulating RVH

- Left axis deviation (item 9c) in 20%

- ST and T wave changes

  - Nonspecific ST and/or T wave abnormalities are common (item 12c)

  - ST and/or T wave changes secondary to ventricular hypertrophy or conduction abnormalities (item 12g)

  - Apical variant of hypertrophic cardiomyopathy has deep T wave inversions in V_4-V_6

- Left atrial abnormality (item 8b) is common; right atrial abnormality (item 8a) on occasion

<u>Note:</u>   The vast majority of patients with hypertrophic cardiomyopathy have abnormal ECGs, with LVH in 50-65%, left atrial abnormality in 20-40%, and pathological Q waves (especially leads I, aVL, V_4 - V_5) in 20-30%. ST and T wave changes (repolarization abnormalities secondary to LVH) are the most common ECG findings, while right axis deviation is rare. Sinus node disease and AV block are occasional manifestations of

this disorder. The most frequent cause of mortality is sudden death, with risk factors including young age and a history of syncope and/or asymptomatic ventricular tachycardia on ambulatory monitoring.

14r. Coronary artery disease

- Use only when definitive evidence of myocardial injury or infarction is present

14s. Central nervous system disorder

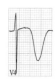

- "Classic changes" of cerebral and subarachnoid hemorrhage usually occur in the precordial leads

  ‣ Large upright or deeply inverted T waves

  ‣ Prolonged QT interval (often marked) (item 12k)

  ‣ Prominent U waves (item 12l)

- Other changes:

  ‣ T wave notching with loss of amplitude

- ▸ ST segment changes:
  - • Diffuse ST elevation mimicking acute pericarditis, *or*
  - • Focal ST elevation mimicking acute myocardial injury, *or*
  - • ST depression
- ▸ Abnormal Q waves mimicking MI
- ▸ Almost any rhythm abnormality (sinus tachycardia or bradycardia, junctional rhythm, VPCs, ventricular tachycardia, etc.)

<u>Note:</u> ECG findings in CNS disease can mimic those of:

- ▸ Acute MI (item 11)
- ▸ Acute pericarditis (item 14p)
- ▸ Drug effect or toxicity (items 14c, d)

14t. Myxedema

- • Low QRS voltage in all leads (item 9b)
- • Sinus bradycardia (item 2c)
- • T wave flattened or inverted
- • PR interval may be prolonged (item 6a)
- • Frequently associated with pericardial effusion (item 14o)
- • Electrical alternans (item 9e) may occur

14u. Hypothermia

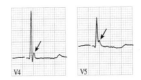

- Sinus bradycardia (item 2a)

- PR, QRS, and QT prolonged (items 2a, 12k)

- Osborne ("J") wave: late upright terminal deflection of QRS complex ("camel hump" sign); amplitude increases as temperature declines

  <u>Note:</u> Notching simulating an Osborne wave may be seen in early repolarization

- Atrial fibrillation (item 2s) in 50-60%

- Other arrhythmias include AV junctional rhythm (item 3d), ventricular tachycardia (item 4f), ventricular fibrillation (item 4i)

14v. Sick sinus syndrome

One or more of the following:

- Marked sinus bradycardia (item 2c)

- Sinus arrest (item 2e) or sinoatrial exit block (item 2f)

- Bradycardia alternating with tachycardia
- Atrial fibrillation with slow ventricular response preceded or followed by sinus bradycardia, sinus arrest, or sinoatrial exit block
- Prolonged sinus node recovery time after atrial premature complex or atrial tachyarrhythmias
- AV junctional escape rhythm
- Additional conduction system disease is often present, including AV block (items 6a-f), IVCD (item 7h), and/or bundle branch block

* * * * *

ECG CRITERIA